MAN AGAINST TSETSE

STRUGGLE FOR AFRICA

MAN AGAINST TSETSE
STRUGGLE FOR AFRICA

JOHN J. McKELVEY, JR.

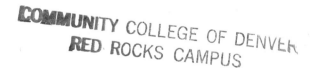

CORNELL UNIVERSITY PRESS

ITHACA AND LONDON

First published 1973 by Cornell University Press.
Published in the United Kingdom by Cornell University Press Ltd.,
2-4 Brook Street, London W1Y 1AA.

International Standard Book Number 0-8014-0768-0
Library of Congress Catalog Card Number 72-12409

Printed in the United States of America by Vail-Ballou Press, Inc.

Librarians: Library of Congress cataloging information
appears on the last page of the book.

To my wife, Jo, who loves books

Preface

The story of the struggle in Africa to overcome the tsetse fly and the diseases it transmits is one of the major epics of man's history; the identification and study of the fly, the discovery of its links to disease in men and animals, the unraveling of how it works its damage, and the campaigns against both the fly and the diseases form major segments of the tale.

This saga represents science at its broadest. It has many heroes, many men groping for truth, making mistakes, finding support and obstacles in bureaucracies, but always building on what other men had found and each contributing in his own way to an arsenal of weapons against a common foe. How man discovers what his biological enemies are, what these mean to him in protecting his own health and in utilizing the natural resources around him, the efforts he feels he must make to combat these enemies, and the constraints that natural laws impose on his efforts to do so are part of this story.

Sleeping sickness in man and nagana in livestock, the diseases transmitted by various species of the tsetse fly, have exerted a tremendous impact on the economic and social development of Africa. Populations of entire villages have been destroyed; the legend of "Negro lethargy" grew up about a people who in fact were suffering from illness; and horses, donkeys, and oxen could not be used to transport men or cargo in many parts of Africa. Missionaries such as David Livingstone, entrepreneurs such as Henry M. Stanley, and colonial governments often found that the fly was one of their chief obstacles. Today, while the tsetse is relatively dormant, new African governments are taking steps to keep it so.

Historians, in dealing with man's relationship with man, too often ignore his relationship with other species in his environment. This history of man's experiences with tsetse shows how men have attempted to cope with the problems caused by an insect and it illustrates how modern economic and medical entomology developed. Entomologists who read this book will find a picture of the evolution of their profession over the past one hundred years. Persons interested in Africa, its people, and its natural resources I hope will gain from this case history an appreciation of the fascinating and difficult biological barriers to progress that Africa has faced.

The narrative that springs from the massive amount of material written about tsetse should have a fullness and a continuity of its own. To help achieve this I have avoided the use of footnotes. Persons wishing to check the accuracy of any detail or interpretation may easily do so by referring to the Bibliographical Essay and Chapter Notes which follow the text and which are coordinated virtually page by page with it. In addition to essential bibliographic data these notes include anecdotes and general observations, some germane to the life and times of the people living and working in Africa during the years that the text covers and others relevant to the story of tsetse, trypanosomes, sleeping sickness, and nagana.

ACKNOWLEDGMENTS

I owe a profound debt of gratitude to The Rockefeller Foundation, which afforded me opportunity in the normal course of my duties to travel widely in Africa and thus to become well acquainted with the problems posed by tsetse flies and the diseases they carry and to come to know the institutions and the people who deal with these problems. I was also able to draw upon the Foundation's library, research, reference, and secretarial resources, and to benefit from a wide variety of other important services. But the views expressed in the text are mine.

In 1963, William C. Cobb, then in charge of the Office of Publications of The Rockefeller Foundation, suggested that I write about the tsetse fly. One of his staff, Elizabeth A. Widenmann, now a librarian at Columbia University, had undertaken research for me on an earlier project; she became my research assistant for this one. The breadth of documentary material used reflects her extensive and persistent search for answers to questions that seemed central to the type of book I wanted to write. The day that she spent with T. A. M. Nash in Bristol was extremely productive, and I am grateful to Dr. Nash for the wealth of information he imparted to her about his life and work on tsetse flies. Members of the staff of the Royal Society of Tropical Medicine and Hygiene kindly made available to her those notes of David Bruce in the Society's possession. Miss Widenmann did a great deal of editorial work on the manuscript; she assembled and drafted the bibliography.

Many of my colleagues have read the manuscript in part or in its entirety. E. C. Stakman, Professor Emeritus of Plant Pathology, University of Minnesota, and Consultant in Agricultural Sciences to The Rockefeller Foundation, for many years followed its progress from the earliest drafts and encouraged me to complete a task that at times, because of the volume of material, seemed insuperable. Wilbur G. Downs, Department of Epidemiology and Public Health, Yale Arbovirus Research Unit, Yale University; John M. Weir, formerly Director of Medical and Natural Sciences, The Rockefeller Foundation, now Consultant, Connecticut Regional Medical Program; John L. Nickel, Associate Director, International Institute of Tropical Agriculture, Ibadan, Nigeria; Carl Koehler, Professor of Entomology, University of California, Berkeley; Ordway Starnes, Director of the Indian Agricultural Program, The Rockefeller Foundation, formerly Director of the East African Agriculture and Forestry Research Organization, Muguga, Kenya; and Thomas R. Odhiambo, Director for Scientific Affairs, The International Centre of Insect Physiology and Ecology, Nairobi, Kenya, were especially helpful. Dr. Nickel, at that time Dean of the Faculty of Agriculture, Makerere University, Kampala, Uganda, submitted the text to B. W. Langlands, Professor of Geography, and to John D. Goodman, Visiting Professor, Department of Agricultural Zoology, Makerere University, who have had a great deal of experience in epidemiology. They checked many of the facts for accuracy and they considered the validity of certain interpretations that I had drawn from them. Montague Yudelman, Senior Advisor, Agriculture Projects Department, International Bank for Reconstruction and Development; William R. Pritchard, Dean, School of Veterinary Medicine, University of California, Davis; Glenn H. Beck, Vice President for Agriculture, Kansas State University; Evelyn W. Nickel; and Eleanor J. B. Starnes also made useful comments.

Several of the most active workers on tsetse flies and African trypanosomiasis offered criticisms and suggestions. J. Fraga de Azevedo reviewed that portion of the manuscript dealing with the Príncipe campaign. Dr. Nash, John F. V. Phillips, and Ernst A. H. Friedheim read the sections of the manuscript relevant to their contributions in the battle against the fly and the diseases it causes. Dr. Phillips, who had worked with C. F. M. Swynnerton, supplied information about him which helped greatly to personalize the account of Swynnerton's life and work with tsetse. Roger J. M. Swynnerton read the material regarding his father's investigations and furnished background details about his father and the portrait of him. Excerpts from the unpublished memoirs of H. C. Stiebel which Mary Stiebel, his daughter-in-law, sent me also added anecdotal material about the elder Swynnerton. Dr. Friedheim in personal conversations broadened my knowledge of the workers in trypanosomiasis research and in action programs of the French-speaking parts of Africa. Thomas Leach, when he was Director of the Nigerian Institute of Trypanosomiasis Research, advised me on certain aspects of tsetse fly research, supplied information about NITR, and arranged to have Alhaji Da'u's photograph taken

Henry Romney, The Rockefeller Foundation's Information Officer, made available facilities and staff expertise of his office; he arranged for outside consultants as well. Muriel Regan, Librarian, and many of her staff, including Marjorie Miller, now with the Fashion Institute of Technology, who undertook a good deal of the interlibrary loan work, facilitated the research in securing books, journals, and other bibliographic items, many of which were difficult to locate. The Chappaqua Library, Chappaqua, New York, also borrowed many books that I needed.

The maps, photographs, and drawings accompanying the text are intended not only to assist the reader in following the story about tsetse and the trypanosomes, but also to make the African setting more vivid. John Morris drew the ten maps. Lonna Lagreco Scott made the drawings of the trypanosomes from live and preserved specimens which William Trager furnished her in his laboratory at Rockefeller University. Elizabeth Muhlfeld of The Rockefeller Foundation's Office of Information assisted in the search for and selection of the photographs. J. K. Crellin, Director of the Wellcome Historical Medical Museum and Library in London, and his staff were extremely helpful.

Most authors, no doubt, are appalled at the number of developmental drafts necessary to bring a manuscript to the point where it logically and clearly expresses their thoughts to the public; this manuscript went through the same process. Charles Pepper, formerly Research Associate, Twentieth Century Fund, took special interest in the book; he worked out a substantial reorganization of the material to emphasize its narrative qualities and to help bring greater sweep and cohesiveness to the story. With unusual patience and understanding combined with technical skill, Susan Hillenbrand, my secretary, bore the responsibility of moving the manuscript from one draft to the next; I am grateful to her especially. I also appreciate the help of Marjorie J. Schad, Program Associate, Patricia Evans, and others of the Foundation staff.

My wife, Josephine Faulkner McKelvey, Young Adult Librarian, Chappaqua Library, gave me the inspiration and encouragement essential to the success of the project. She spent many hours editing, checking quotations, and verifying citations to ensure that a researcher, using this book as a sound initial source, can probe deeply into many aspects of the biology and control of tsetse flies and trypanosomes. Aided by Terrill R. McKelvey, she compiled the index. I am deeply grateful to her for her assistance.

JOHN J. McKELVEY, JR.

New York City

Contents

Illustrations

TABLE

MAN AGAINST TSETSE

STRUGGLE FOR AFRICA

I

The Curse of Flies

And then, there were the flies. They swarmed everywhere, and persecuted the Family all day long. They were the first animals up, in the morning, and the last ones down, at night. But they must not be killed, they must not be injured, they were sacred, their origin was divine, they were the special pets of the Creator, his darlings.

Mark Twain
Letters from the Earth

Walk over the stubble of the cereal crops teff and wheat in the highlands of Ethiopia during the dry season. Hordes of small face flies coming up stealthily from nowhere will cluster around your mouth and eyes. Their unmerciful attack will drive you to the shade of the eucalyptus trees, where they are unlikely to follow. Or drive along the dusty tracks and trails in the Rift Valley in Kenya and watch the tall, lordly Masai people. You will see these flies thick on their faces, feeding on the mucus of their lips and eyes. The scantily clad, spear-bearing Masai have long since given up brushing the flies away, and somehow they seem to coexist comfortably with flies on their bodies and around their thorny twig corrals. These face flies belong to the same family as the common housefly; their mouth parts are spongy, and they do not bite in the true sense of the word. Apparently they do not nourish and transmit a specific disease as some other flies do. But mechanically, by picking up

1

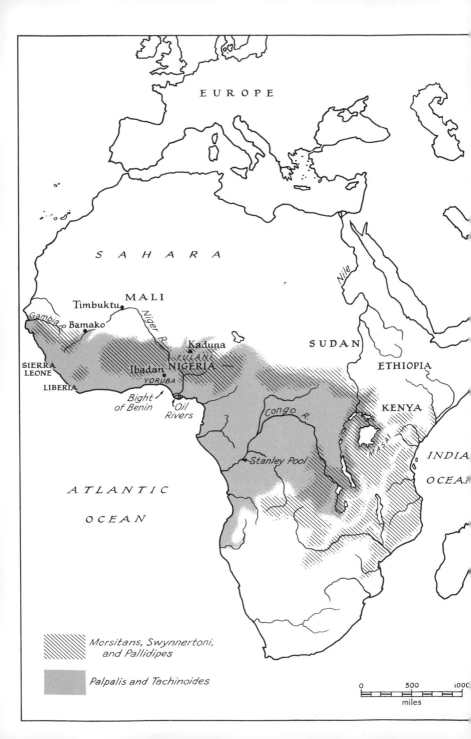

a tiny organism from one victim and leaving it with the next, they spread the blinding disease trachoma.

Submit, if you like, to the annoyance of clouds of stocky black flies that bite in the fullest sense of the word. In parts of southern Sudan during seasons when these flies are numerous, tribal people may carry, even wear, smoldering masses of rope to fend them off with smoke. Born of fast-flowing streams and rapids, these black flies process through their systems the tiny threadworms that infect people with river blindness.

Or take a local plane from Kaduna to Ibadan in Nigeria. On the seat in front of you may rest a fellow passenger, a big, brownish fly with a long, thin snout. Or tramp through the tall grass around thornbush in an East African lowland, the Manyara Game Park, for example, and stir up legions of similar flies from a spot where animals have lain. This is the tsetse, which will attack you with relish and will infect you, if you are unlucky, with a wasting disease called human trypanosomiasis, or sleeping sickness.

So insidious is this disease, so benign, apparently, the early symptoms, that one really has to exercise his imagination to decide whether or not he has it. It starts with a simple red swelling at the site of a tsetse bite. Malaise, lassitude, and low-grade fever lasting off and on for two years may ensue. Insomnia at night, drowsiness during the daytime, and headache constitute some of the observable symptoms. Soon after the onset of the disease a rash may appear, especially around the trunk, chest, and back; brought out sometimes after hot baths, this rash appears at irregular intervals. Muscular cramps and neurological pains become common. Swollen glands are another symptom.

These symptoms coupled with others occurring in the right progression spell sleeping sickness as a disease and death to the victim. The fever accompanied by a fast pulse develops with a rigor and severe sweating, especially at night. Generalized puf-

of Africa showing distribution of tsetse species. (Drawn by John Morris.)

finess of the face, which gives the features a rather inane chubby expression, develops. Daytime drowsiness and nocturnal sleeplessness increase. Malnutrition sets in because the sleepiness eventually becomes so overpowering that the patient does not take food unless aroused. He loses interest in his surroundings, is unable to concentrate even on minor matters, grows irritable, melancholy, emotional, depressed; his memory fades, and his intelligence and character disintegrate until he finally becomes comatose and dies.

The tsetse and other flies, deadly or no more than a nuisance, still constitute a significant problem in Africa despite the weapons in hand to battle them. When most people think of Africa they think of the savannas teeming with exotic game they have seen in movies and on television or, if they are older, they may remember the dark, hostile setting of the yarns of Edgar Rice Burroughs and H. Rider Haggard. Anyone who has been there knows that the continent is very different from this. Its capitals are as modern and bustling as any in the world, its leaders are searching with vigor and intelligence for ways to modernize their lands, and some of its best-known game species are in danger of vanishing forever. But in many places in this beautiful land the visitor from any urban area is struck by the abundance of flies. Even tsetse still abounds, though it has been the target of one of the broadest and most intensive eradication campaigns in history. Its numbers have been reduced, and in most places its diseases are less feared for the moment. But it thrives in grasslands and forests and river courses, and it still kills several thousand people a year. As long as it lives and kills a few, it is a danger. If lapses in attention to tsetse occur, it is capable of sapping the vitality of large numbers of people who need all their energy and resources for the difficult task of development.

Just as sleeping sickness and other health problems hamper

the development of sub-Saharan Africa today, so they must have in the remote past. Many blank pages in European as well as in African history block our search for knowledge of the origins of this disease and its effects; early observations were often imprecise and symptoms of the disease were easily confused with those of other illnesses, so that we cannot identify any early description of an illness as sleeping sickness.

Nevertheless the disease was surely present in West Africa and the Congo basin for centuries. Ibn Khaldun, an Arabian historian, reported that a disease which may have been sleeping sickness commonly affected those of the higher classes in the Mali kingdom during the fourteenth century, when it reached its zenith as the richest and most powerful empire of the western Sudan, an empire which built its capital along the Niger River upstream from Bamako, capital of modern Mali. One of its kings, Mansa Djata, suffered from this disease for two years, then died of it in 1374. The description of his illness as recounted by a local man of proven veracity leaves little doubt that he really had sleeping sickness. Nearly five hundred years later the disease still seemed to be affecting people of the higher classes. In Liberia the African scholar Doalu Bukere contracted a disease that apparently was sleeping sickness. Fortunately, assisted by five of his friends, he was able to complete his alphabet in Vai for his people before at age forty he died of this illness in 1850.

Some students believe that at one time the disease existed only in West Africa and in the Congo basin. Others think that the disease organism was present in many other places as well and that only the absence of the right number of people with the right sorts of habits in connection with the right distribution of flies prevented wider incidence of sickness.

It is also certain that an animal disease we now know is related, commonly called nagana or tsetse-fly disease, was much more widespread. While it did not seem seriously to affect the wild animals abundant in Africa's forests and grasslands, it afflicted domestic animals, notably cattle and horses. In certain areas cattle could thrive, and Africans founded whole social orders on the possession of cattle. But the number of such places was limited, and horses and oxen could never be used for transportation across the disease-ridden rivers and valleys between disease-free pockets.

In the fifteenth century, Henry the Navigator and his Portuguese seamen, looking for a shortcut to the source of West African gold, sailed up the River Gambia and came upon the local people engaged in the "silent trade," an honor system of exchanging gold for salt and other commodities which northerners brought south across the Sahara by caravan. The northerners would display their wares in the marketplace silently and then disappear. The local people would lay out a quantity of gold and likewise retreat. Barter would continue in this fashion until the price was right. Trading took place in the region of Wangara, a name which time has obliterated from modern maps but which was an area of present-day Mali bordering the forested zone to the east and south and the desert to the north and west. The caravan leaders of the Sahara guided their animals just so far and no farther into the humid, forested zone for fear their animals might come down with disease and die, bitten by tsetse.

The early growth of one of the largest inland cities of black Africa, Ibadan in present-day Nigeria, may be due in large part to the presence of the fly. The Yorubas and other peoples of the humid south could not keep horses because of fly disease. In the mid-1800's, Fulani cavalry sweeping south tried to capture Ibadan and other Yoruba cities bordering the savanna area occupied by the Fulani; they failed because they lost great military advantage when their horses came down with the disease transmitted by tsetse. However, they ravaged the Yoruba settlements in the savanna lands to the north, and refugees retreated to Ibadan to swell the population of that city.

In spite of the presence of disease, Africans developed significant cultures, as shown by their achievements in music and the sophistication of their art in such centers as Benin. But when one considers the contribution of animal power to the development of Europe and Asia, it is safe to conclude that its absence handicapped Africa enormously.

One of the first medical observations of sleeping sickness was reported by John Atkins, a surgeon in the British navy. Early in the history of the slave trade, slavers learned to identify victims of what was called "Negro lethargy" among slave cargoes and to avoid persons with swollen neck glands, a common early symptom. Atkins served on these slave ships between West Africa and the West Indies in the 1720's and 1730's and recorded his observations. He noticed that the afflicted slaves would experience a loss of appetite two or three days before the onset of drowsiness. He wrote:

Their Sleeps are sound, and Sense of Feeling very little; for pulling, drubbing, or whipping, will scarce stir up Sense and Power enough to move; and the Moment you cease beating, the Smart is forgot, and down they fall again into a State of Insensibility, drivling constantly from the Mouth, as if in a deep Salivation; breath slowly, but not unequally, nor snort.

According to Atkins, the young contracted the "Sleepy Distemper" more readily than the old; those from the country got it more frequently than those from the coast.

Atkins believed the immediate and basic cause of "Sleepy Distemper" to be a superabundance of phlegm pouring out from the brain. He ascribed "Negro lethargy" to the common cold, to a long period of immaturity of the African, to a poor and indiscriminate diet and way of life, and to a natural weakness of the brain. These causes interacted with one another, he thought. He considered weakness of the brain the most important cause, a weakness brought about by lack of use. Atkins went on to propose remedies typical of his day—among them, bleeding of the jugular vein, quick purges, using snuff, and applying blister-producing substances. He also recommended sudden plunges into the sea.

For prevention or cure of sleepy distemper, Atkins' prescriptions were worthless; so were his conceptions of the causes. But they did epitomize the thinking of his time about the people of Africa, and they demonstrated a dislike and a rejection of a foreign culture. They were tantamount to a curse in the African sense of the word, one that stuck for generations—an inference of stupidity, inferiority, ineptness, weakness, and disease. This curse prevailed throughout Africa's colonial period, until the unfolding of knowledge brought a true understanding of the disease and its cause.

Some hundred years after Atkins' recommendations for dunking victims of sleeping sickness in the sea, a curious fly from the Congo came into the possession of a French collector. How it got to him, no one knows, but it may have been caught by John Cranch, collector of objects of natural history on a disastrous British scientific expedition in 1816.

Cranch was a self-taught naturalist. He showed intelligence and industry at an early age; his penurious guardian apprenticed him as a shoemaker. Nevertheless he refused to suppress his interest in natural history, and he devoted every spare moment to reading and collecting. As a youth, his biographer tells us, "he was able to draw up correct and classical descriptions of all the insects he could procure in the neighbourhood of Kingsbridge."

In time he was able to set up his own shop, and leaving shoe-making to his journeymen he threw himself into his interests. His writing and collecting attracted the attention of scientists at the British Museum, who set him to gathering marine speci-mens on the coast of Devon and Cornwall. He responded by discovering an "infinity of new objects." When the Admiralty decided to fit an expedition to the Congo River, Cranch was of-fered a post and immediately accepted.

The expedition was led by Commander James Kingston Tuckey, a hero of the Napoleonic wars. Its main purpose was geographic. The British entertained a theory that the Niger River, known as the major stream of West Africa's interior since Roman times, found its outlet in the Congo. A German theory that its outlet was the Oil Rivers, an often-visited delta with many mouths on the Bight of Benin, was scoffed at. (In 1830 Richard and John Lander proved this theory correct.) The expedition was therefore to trace the Congo to its source to see if it was the same stream that flowed past fabled Timbuktu. Another expedition was planned to cross to the Niger overland and follow it downstream. An earlier explorer, Mungo Park, had tried this in 1805 and had disappeared after reporting that all but ten of his thirty-nine companions had died of fever.

But the Congo expedition was also charged with gathering information on the animal and plant life, the minerals, the cli-mate, and the people it came across. To do this, a botanist also skilled in geology, a comparative anatomist, and a specialist from the Royal Garden at Kew were added to the expedition. From the way the British and other colonial powers used such information in other times and places, probably an unstated motive for these instructions was commercial and imperial ex-ploitation. But a pure thirst for knowledge played an important role too. As Dr. John Douglas said in an introduction to an account of Cook's third voyage: "Indeed, it would argue a most culpable want of rational curiosity, if we did not use our best endeavours to arrive at a full acquaintance with the contents of our own planet."

The expedition found the climate of the Congo equable and the country "remarkably free from teazing and noxious insects." Nevertheless many of its members were quickly stricken by disease, and even the strongest explored little farther than halfway to Stanley Pool. Except for the gardener, the entire professional staff was wiped out; of fifty-six persons who started out on the expedition, twenty-one died, including Tuckey and Cranch. Some apparently died of yellow fever, the mosquito-borne disease already known in the West Indies; others "appeared to have no other ailment than that which had been caused by extreme fatigue, and actually to have died from exhaustion." Their fate was attributed not to insect bites but to the Congo water.

Nevertheless some of Cranch's specimens arrived in Britain. Of the insects, "thirty-six species only reached England in a tolerable state, the rest were entirely destroyed by insects and damp." Whether one of these thirty-six was the fly that found its way into the Frenchman's collection can only be left to conjecture; but no other systematic collecting in the Congo Basin is known before this time.

The state of biological science in Cranch's day may seem crude to a modern reader. At a time when French and British warships could blast one another with twenty-four-pound cannon in any waters of the world, the ignorance was appalling. But science was yet young, and Cranch's enthusiasm for collecting represented a stage it had to go through before it could make further advances. In all areas of biology the aim was to discover and to classify. Linnaeus, the great Swedish botanist who died in 1778, had provided the key. Some plants and animals could be seen to resemble others closely enough to be re-

garded as kin, but to differ in specific ways. Houseflies and
fruit flies are an example. More distant kinship could then be
discerned in still more unlike creatures such as houseflies and
mosquitoes. Thus the whole of life could be fitted into two trees
of which the trunks were the plant and animal kingdoms and the
smallest twigs the innumerable species. Tsetse flies today are
classed as a genus in the order Diptera, which includes midges
and mosquitoes, and the family Muscoidea, which includes houseflies. The tsetse genus is broken down into twenty-one or
twenty-two species. In all there are some 80,000 different species of flies, and more are identified every year.

The fly that may have been caught by Cranch first turned up
in the collection of an especially colorful character in the history of entomology, Count Pierre François Aimé Auguste Dejean (1780–1845). A "General of the Empire and Aide-de-
camp to Napoleon I . . . he never lost a chance to add [an
insect] to his collection   At the battle of Alcanizas [in
Spain], which Dejean won after a very hard fight in which he
took a great number of prisoners, he suddenly saw near a little
brook a brilliant and rare" beetle resting on a flower. "At the
head of his troops, facing the enemy," Count Dejean "was
about to give the signal to charge, but, seeing the insect, he at
once dismounted, captured it, pinned it in his helmet, re-
mounted his horse, and gave the order for one of the most vigorous charges of the campaign. After the battle he found that
his helmet had been 'horriblement maltraité' by a cannon-ball,"
but he recovered his precious beetle intact.

All of the soldiers in his regiment learned to collect insects.
Each carried a small vial of alcohol in which to place the insects he collected. Even the enemy knew of Dejean's "eccentric-
ity." "Those who found dead soldiers on the field having with
them a little bottle containing insects in alcohol" always carried
the bottle to Dejean, regardless of who won the battle.

The count's mysterious fly was examined by a French entomologist, André Jean Baptiste Robineau-Desvoidy, who in
1830 published a study entitled *Essai sur les Myodaires* in which
he described a fly he said came from the Congo. He assigned it
the generic name *Nemorhina,* meaning thread-nosed, and the
specific name *palpalis,* which refers to the prominent sheaths of
the long tubular sucking organ of the fly, its proboscis. In his
description he surmised that the slender proboscis, or snout,
was too frail to cause damage.

The genus name *Nemorhina* never took hold, partly perhaps
because someone lost Robineau-Desvoidy's type specimen. Even
such a sleuth of the dead flies as Major Ernest Edward Austen,
who published the first major monograph on tsetse in 1903,
could not turn it up after an exhaustive search. In the late
1830's, Count Dejean, then approaching sixty and troubled
with failing eyesight, disposed of his collection to various buy-
ers. It seems likely that the Diptera—including the *Nemorhina*
type specimen—were acquired by another French entomologist,
J. M. F. Bigot, who was then beginning his work with flies. But
Bigot was a very sloppy entomologist indeed. He had the dangerous habit of removing the original labels from the pinned insect specimens he received and of copying the locality information onto new labels, which he placed in the boxes with them.
He introduced thereby the chance of associating specimens with
the wrong labels. For example, he described one species as
Glossina ventricosa; this got mixed in with some flies that came
from Australia—so he assumed that *G. ventricosa* came from
Australia. Actually his specimen was a dead tsetse of the species identified by Robineau-Desvoidy but with its abdomen engorged with coagulated blood. Thus it did not stand as a new
species, much less as coming from Australia. Ultimately the
Dejean flies probably reached G. H. Verrall, who bought the
Bigot collection. When Austen borrowed this material from

Verrall he found no trace of Robineau-Desvoidy's type specimen. It might have been among the unlabeled ones, but in that case its identification was gone forever.

The honor of giving the tsetse fly the scientific name it bears today went instead to Dr. Christian Rudolf Wilhelm Wiedemann, a German entomologist, zoologist, and medical doctor. Wiedemann's specimen came from the collection of the Swedish entomologist, Carl Friedrich Fallén. It had been collected by Adam Afzelius, a Swedish naturalist and student of Linnaeus, when he had served as botanist with the Sierra Leone Company in 1792–1796 in a project to revive the English-backed settlement of freed slaves that had failed earlier. Wiedemann, a professor at the University of Kiel, named the fly *Glossina longipalpis* (tongue fly with the long tasting organ) in his monumental *Aussereuropaische zweiflügelige Insekten* (Two-winged Insects outside Europe), also published in 1830. This designation stuck; all species of tsctse flies now bear the generic name *Glossina*. Following scientific tradition, the *longipalpis* species became the type specimen for the genus, though it is not as much of a threat to man or animals as several others. The later specimens, like men lined up behind the leader of a marching band, were supposed to be more or less true to type.

In southern Africa, though sleeping sickness was unknown, a devastating disease later identified as nagana afflicted domestic livestock. But here, unlike the tribes to the north, Africans saw a link between the tsetse fly and the disease, probably because the species of fly living here could not survive everywhere but existed in scattered pockets that fluctuated and shifted with the seasons. When the fly's numbers thinned out, people could maintain their cattle with relative impunity. During some seasons, the fly might be virtually nonexistent or, if present, it would be rare enough so that they would lose only a few cattle

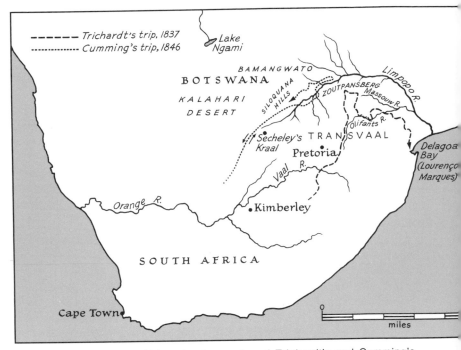

Map of southern Africa showing routes of Trichardt's and Cumming's trips. (Drawn by John Morris.)

at a time. The fluctuations between light and heavy infestations gave the people a basis of comparison enabling them to discover why some stock got by and other stock did not. This knowledge of the fly's effect on cattle helped them to prepare modes of attack against it. Herding cattle into fly-free areas, shooting out game in infested areas, and destroying tsetse's favorite resting and breeding sites were all methods employed to combat the outbreak of nagana.

The first white men to occupy the Transvaal were the Voortrekkers, the farmers of Dutch descent who moved from the

Cape area to the Transvaal in the 1830's to escape British domination and later founded a state there. They were forced to plan their routes to avoid the fly. In 1837, Louis Trichardt, a noted Voortrekker, led a party numbering about fifty from their isolated and troubled two-year-old settlement at Zoutpansberg near the Limpopo River toward Delagoa Bay (Lourenço Marques). The subleader of the party was Jan Pretorius, a member of the famous South African Boer family. The party wanted to go due east, but the native people persuaded them not to because of the fly on the Massouw River. Instead they detoured south along the Olifants River, crossing it at thirteen different places. But they came to a cul-de-sac—a valley with mountain barriers on three sides—and there met a swarm of tsetse that bit their oxen and decimated them.

At least twice along the journey, Trichardt's eighteen-year-old son, Pieta, caught a tsetse in his hands; he showed a crushed one to Jan Pretorius. Neither recognized it for what it really was. Perhaps they thought it to be an extraordinary housefly. Upon arrival at Delagoa Bay, the expedition collapsed; all but one of its male members died of malaria.

A hunter from Scotland also met difficulty with the fly in South Africa in the mid-1840's. He was Roualeyn Gordon Cumming, who early in life had acquired a love of natural history and of sport, but after finishing his education at Eton he sailed for India to join his regiment in 1839. He disliked the Indian climate, so he returned home as soon as possible to indulge in deer stalking, his favorite pastime. He quickly tired of hunting in Scotland, "where the game was strictly preserved, and where the continual presence of keepers and foresters took away half the charm of the chase." In 1843 he obtained a commission as a Cape Rifleman in South Africa, but with no fighting in prospect he promptly bought his way out of the army and turned to hunting in the interior.

Cumming plied the hunting grounds and the tributaries of

the Limpopo, which Rudyard Kipling later crossed when Cecil Rhodes sent him north to Bulawayo to see the province now Rhodesia, and which he immortalized as the "great grey-green, greasy Limpopo River, all set about with fever-trees" in "The Elephant's Child," one of the *Just So Stories*. Cumming rode horseback and used oxen to pull his wagons. The ivory he collected paid for his expeditions, but his overriding interest was in collecting hunting trophies and objects of interest in science and natural history.

On one occasion, Cumming went from the highland area of Bamangwato down to the hunting grounds of the Limpopo against the advice of the local people, the Tswanas. They had told him that Moselekatze, the fierce Matabele chief, would probably seize his property and murder him if he hunted in the Limpopo lowlands. At the very least, he would lose all his horses and oxen to a fly called tsetse. Moselekatze neither murdered him nor confiscated his property, but tsetse did attack his horses, one of which died.

On another trip to the lowlands, Cumming reported:

I met with the famous fly called "tsetse," whose bite is certain death to oxen and horses . . . ; they are very quick and active, and storm a horse like a swarm of bees, alighting on him in hundreds and drinking his blood. The animal thus bitten pines away and dies at periods varying from a week to three months, according to the extent to which he has been bitten.

Though he fled from the fly pocket, all his stock began to waste and die. "The cattle presented a most woeful appearance," he wrote. "Listless and powerless, they cared not to feed, and, though the grass covered the country with the richest and most luxuriant pasturage, their sides remained hollow, and their whole bodies became daily more emaciated; the eyes also of many of them were closed and swollen." Cumming dispatched a messenger with a sealed bottle containing a note to a friend, the young missionary doctor David Livingstone, at the kraal of Sechele, a famous Tswana chief in the highlands. Livingstone sent new trek oxen to Cumming so that he could complete his trip and return to the highlands.

"Tsetse" was the fly's name among the Tswana people along the border of the Kalahari Desert, who also used the term to designate the fly's buzz. The Tswana probably occupied the fly country of the Cameroon several hundred years ago, but militant tribes from the north drove them far south to Botswana, where they live today.

Africans in other areas used different names for the fly. The Ethiopians called it "tsaltsalya," as they did all bloodsucking pests. The Hausa of the Niger country named it "tsande," which, with its "ts," may echo the "music" the fly makes when preening itself at rest. Certain others referred to it as "nsinsi," perhaps in imitation of its high pitched pinging sound, which may be a mating call. Austen thought the name "tsetse" was a corruption of "nsinsi."

Cumming, in any case, picked up the name "tsetse" from the Tswana. His use of it in his popular book *Five Years of a Hunter's Life in the Far Interior of Africa,* first published in 1850, established the name in the English language.

Others in transit to or from India or other countries where they held army commissions or colonial posts used to stop for furlough at the cape in South Africa to hunt in the same general locality as did Cumming. Among the visitors were Captain (later Major) Frank Vardon of the Madras Army and William Cotton Oswell. "I will not attempt to describe him," Oswell wrote about Vardon. "Let every man picture for himself the most perfect fellow-traveller he can imagine, and that's Frank." Oswell, with Livingstone and Mungo Murray, was one of the discoverers of Lake Ngami in Botswana. Livingstone became a mailbox link between the colonial and army officers in India and those in Africa. Once when Cumming came down with malaria in Africa, and did not do so well in collecting trophies, Oswell found out about it in India through a letter from Livingstone.

Oswell and Vardon met the tsetse in 1845 while hunting on the low Siloquana Hills near the Limpopo. Oswell described the fly as a "dusky-grey, long-winged, vicious-looking fly," two or three of which would kill the largest ox or strongest horse. He wrote:

We examined about twenty of our beasts after death, and the appearances were similar in all—flesh flaccid and offensive, fat, if any remained, like yellow water, membrane between skin and flesh suffused with lymph, and puffy, stomach and intestines healthy, heart and liver, and occasionally lungs diseased. The heart in particular attracted our attention. It was no longer a firm muscle, but flabby, like flesh steeped in water, blood gelatinous and scanty. . . . The fly infests particular spots, from which it *never* shifts. The natives herd their cattle at a distance from its haunts, and should they . . . be obliged to pass through tracts of country in which it exists, they choose a moonlight winter's night, as during the nights of the cold season it does not bite.

Vardon on this hunting trip decided to make sure that the fly and not some poisonous plant caused the disease. He rode a horse into a fly pocket, let it be bitten, caught several fly specimens, and rode out again without permitting the horse to graze. Vardon later gave the flies to Dr. John Obadiah Westwood, an entomologist in London. "The specimens you saw," he wrote the scientist later, "cost me one of the best [horses] in my stud."

Westwood identified the fly as a new species of *Glossina,* which he named *morsitans* (biting). He reported his observations to the Zoological Society in 1850. Curiously, Westwood's drawing of a typical specimen contained a serious error. Somehow the head had been torn from the thorax and had been glued back on in the wrong position. Westwood's drawing faithfully reproduced this defect. The figure, mistake and all, was reproduced on the title page of Livingstone's *Missionary Travels and Researches in South Africa* in 1857. Westwood later complained that the drawing was borrowed without permission, but Livingstone's transgression was apparently unintentional.

Hunters like Cumming, Oswell, and Vardon came and went with the seasons; David Livingstone spent thirty-two years in Africa. All were afflicted with a wanderlust that drove them deeper into tsetse fly country than Europeans had ever penetrated before. In the hunters, the wanderlust was fueled by the lure of big game and adventure. Livingstone, however, was driven by a thirst to spread Christianity and to enlarge geographical knowledge. And since, as he said, "the end of the geographical feat is but the beginning of missionary enterprise," perhaps his religion was the greater motive.

From the start of his career in Africa in 1841, however, Livingstone's missionary philosophy was different from that of his future father-in-law, the Reverend Robert Moffat, and most other missionaries of the time. Moffat built one mission station at Kuruman, Bechuanaland, South Africa, and spent his entire career there. Most of his colleagues did likewise. Livingstone, on the other hand, believed it was better to train local people to take over the mission work in a given spot and then to establish another station elsewhere. A physician, he also believed that it was important to look after the health of men's bodies as well as their souls, and he regarded the esteem his medicine brought him as an important asset in his evangelism.

In time he came to believe that Africa had to be "civilized" in order to Christianize it. He saw poverty, ignorance, aspects

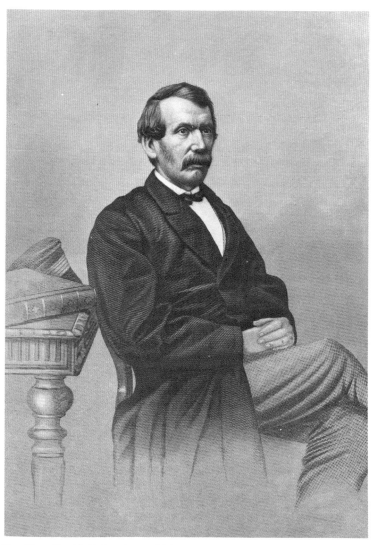

The Rev. David Livingstone, African traveler and missionary. (Engraving, The Bettmann Archive.)

of tribalism, and above all the hated Portuguese and Arabic slave trade as the greatest evils in African society. The Africans, he believed, were not a "fallen" but a "suffering" people. To improve their life he thought in terms of giving them access to "legitimate" commerce, producing and selling cotton, for example, to replace slave trading and similar evils. In the last part of his career, no longer formally a missionary, he devoted his energies to this end.

Livingstone's ideas were radically different from those of other Protestant missionaries and theologians of his day. But they revolutionized missionary operations and attracted missionaries to Africa in the years that followed. Many of these men and women had to deal directly, in a pragmatic way, with the health and suffering of people afflicted with sleeping sickness where that disease broke out in epidemic proportions.

Livingstone was born in Blantyre, Scotland, in 1813 and was sent to work in a cotton mill at the age of ten. His thirst for broader horizons, however, made him a constant reader, on the job and off; his favorite subjects were science and travel and, at his father's insistence, religion. Persuading his father to let him study medicine (which was difficult, for his father thought him motivated by greed), he entered Anderson's University in Glasgow in 1836 and studied chemistry, medicine, and theology.

In 1840, Livingstone qualified in medicine and was ready for a mission under the sponsorship of the nonsectarian London Missionary Society. He wanted to go to China, where a few medical missionaries had gained entrance, but the Opium War made this impossible and he was persuaded by Moffat, then visiting Britain, to go to South Africa. After a time at Kuruman, Livingstone established his own station at Kolobeng, 270 miles away. In 1845 he married Moffat's oldest daughter, Mary.

But he grew restless here and saw the proximity of the Boers

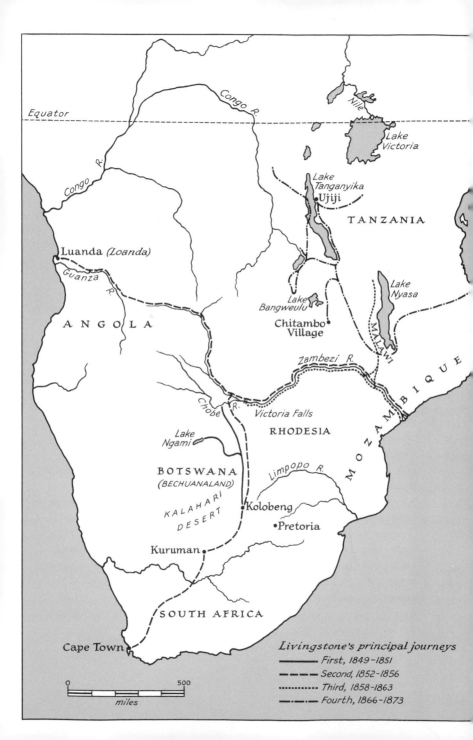

Equator

Congo R.

Congo R.

Nile

Lake
Victoria

Lake
Tanganyika
Ujiji

T A N Z A N I A

Luanda (Loanda)

Guanza R.

A N G O L A

Lake
Nyasa

Lake
Bangweulu

Chitambo
Village

M A L A W I

Zambezi R.

Chobe R.

Victoria Falls

M O Z A M B I Q U E

Lake
Ngami

R H O D E S I A

Limpopo R.

B O T S W A N A
(BECHUANALAND)

K A L A H A R I
D E S E R T

Kolobeng

•Pretoria

Kuruman

S O U T H   A F R I C A

Cape Town

0   500
miles

Livingstone's principal journeys
———— *First, 1849-1851*
– – – – *Second, 1852-1856*
·············· *Third, 1858-1863*
–·–·–·– *Fourth, 1866-1873*

as a hindrance to his scheme of native evangelism. This led him to explore the land to the north in four trips, in 1849, 1850, 1851, and 1866. On his first trip accompanied by Oswell and Mungo Murray, both sportsmen, he crossed the Kalahari Desert and reached Lake Ngami. His wife and three children accompanied him on his second and third trips; Oswell also went with him on the third trip.

In 1852, having sent his family to Britain, he set out north from Cape Town and reached the Zambezi River near the point where the boundaries of Botswana, Zambia, and Rhodesia come together. Accompanied by the traditional African guides and bearers but by no white men, he followed the river upstream and continued westward to Luanda (Loanda) in Portuguese Angola. Then, refusing passage to England, he retraced his path and followed the Zambezi to its mouth in Mozambique, discovering Victoria Falls on the way. The journey took four years.

News of his travels aroused great enthusiasm in England, and when he returned there in December 1856 he was acclaimed as a national hero. Though Portuguese explorers had traveled extensively in the interior of southern Africa before Livingstone, their accounts were largely unknown in Britain. His *Missionary Travels and Researches in South Africa,* published in 1857, enjoyed a wide sale. With his new perspective on his mission in Africa he resigned from the London Missionary Society and in 1858 returned to Africa as a British consul.

In the following years he explored Lake Nyasa and the rivers emptying into the sea on the lower east coast. He thought white colonization in the highlands would help destroy the slave trade and establish Christianity. But there was dissension among the white members of his expeditions, and, a cruel blow, his wife, who rejoined him in 1862, died three months later. Recalled by the British government in 1863, he first sailed to Bombay in a

of Africa showing David Livingstone's travels. (Drawn by John Morris.)

steamship he had hoped to install on Lake Nyasa, arrived in Britain in 1864, and there wrote his second book, *Narrative of an Expedition to the Zambesi and Its Tributaries.*

His last series of explorations occupied him from 1866 till his death. Obsessed with finding unknown headwaters of the Nile, he explored Lake Tanganyika and what were later determined to be the headwaters of the Congo. "The Nile sources," he wrote, "are valuable to me only as a means of enabling me to open my mouth with power among men. It is this power I hope to apply to remedy an enormous evil [the slave trade]." It was in 1871, when he was thought to have disappeared, that he had his famous encounter with Henry Morton Stanley in the village of Ujiji. Two years later he died at Chitambo's village south of Lake Bangweulu, apparently of rectal bleeding; a suggestion that he died of sleeping sickness is not credited.

Livingstone's travels frequently brought him into contact with *Glossina morsitans* and at least two other species of tsetse; his writings are sprinkled with descriptions of these encounters. He paid heed when the local people pointed out fly pockets, and when he had to cross them with horses or oxen he did so at night, for the fly bit only during the daytime. He had learned that the fly was associated with game, particularly buffalo, and he feared that buffalo might have brought the fly into certain areas he had to cross. As a result, when he saw buffalo he walked ahead of his party by day and his men brought up the oxen and wagons by night. He, and Oswell too, recognized a close association of the fly with elephants. The Portuguese whom Livingstone met in Mozambique also noted this association; they called the tsetse the elephant fly.

Despite his caution, however, Livingstone often lost oxen to the fly. On his second journey north from Kolobeng he spent four days in the Kalahari Desert without finding water. On finding a rhinoceros trail he unyoked the oxen, which rushed to a

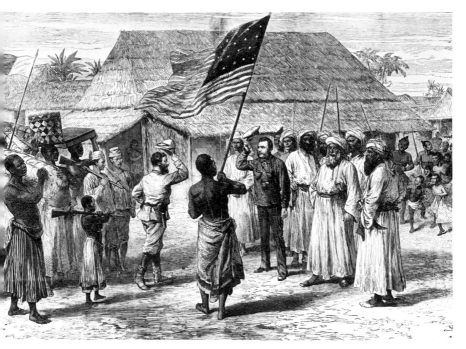

Stanley meeting with Livingstone at Ujiji, Lake Tanganyika. "The engraving, for which I supplied the materials is as correct as if the scene had been photographed," Stanley said. (Engraving, The Bettmann Archive.)

river some distance away. On the way they crossed a small patch of trees containing tsetse. This and other encounters cost him forty-three oxen on this trip. On his transcontinental trek his favorite ox, Sinbad, which had carried him a considerable distance, was badly bitten despite his having detailed a man with a branch to ward off the flies as they went along. A day later Sinbad developed spots with patches of hair a half-inch broad wetted by exudation where the flies had bitten. Livingstone and his men first thought about slaughtering and eating the ox to allay their hunger for meat, but they decided to put him out to pasture and let him end his days in peace. Shortly afterward Sinbad succumbed to tsetse fly disease.

But though the flies frequently bit Livingstone and his companions on their travels, they were never blamed for a human illness. He described how one took a meal out of the back of his hand. It inserted deep into his flesh the middle prong of the three parts of its proboscis, then drew it out slightly. A pool of blood formed, and the proboscis assumed a crimson color as the mandibles went into brisk operation. The fly's previously shrunken belly swelled. When the fly was satisfied it quietly departed. The bite left a slight itchy irritation but virtually no inflammation. He could have agreed with Vardon, who said the bite of the tsetse felt like a flea bite.

Once he thought he had a tsetse imprisoned in his shirt pocket. But it buzzed around loose underneath his shirt during the night and found its way to his stomach. Three red spots showed on his skin in the morning, each about an inch in diameter. He noticed local uneasiness, pain, and itch combined, but he thought the sensation was less bothersome than a mosquito bite.

Where game had been eliminated, the fly seemed less prevalent than in areas heavily populated with game. In the former areas cattle did well, but in the latter ones people kept goats, not cattle, on account of the abundance of the fly. Livingstone assumed that the goats must be immune to fly disease. He decided that game animals affected by fly bite, like goats, might also be immune. Goats are not, in fact, immune, but they do manifest high tolerance to some forms of the disease in some areas. Most wild game also appear to be highly tolerant.

An alternative to the constant loss of horses and oxen seemed to Livingstone to be to import water buffalo from India and camels from the desert countries in North Africa. Such animals might possess a high degree of resistance, if not immunity, to the fly disease. Livingstone brought in water buffalo and camels following a visit to India in 1866, but, alas, in due course these animals came down with tsetse fly disease. Bent on proving his hunch a good one—that they would be immune—he stubbornly clung to the belief they had died of other causes, when in his heart he knew better.

A keen observer, Livingstone watched an insect predator, a robber fly of the family Asilidae, long-legged and gaunt-looking, alight on the bare ground, spring upon tsetse and other flies, suck out their blood, and throw the bodies away. Unfortunately, too few robber flies attack tsetse to turn the predator into a useful biological means for controlling the tsetse fly population. Livingstone may also have been the first to observe the relationship between the bite of a tick and relapsing fever, a disease afflicting human beings in Africa and other continents.

In his first book Livingstone inserted a careful description of *G. morsitans* and its effects. It differed little from those of earlier travelers, but the physician in him led him to speculate on how the little fly could kill such mighty animals. "These symptoms seem to indicate," he wrote, "what is probably the case, a poison in the blood, the germ of which enters when the proboscis is inserted to draw blood. The poison-germ, contained in a bulb at the root of the proboscis, seems capable, although very minute in quantity, of reproducing itself, for the blood after death by tsetse is very small in quantity, and scarcely stains the hands in dissection." Though the statement does not point to a living organism as the cause of the sickness, it is remarkable for the time, since the germ theory of disease had hardly been put forward then and was not firmly established by Louis Pasteur until 1861.

Livingstone also experimented with arsenic as a cure for

tsetse fly disease. The idea might have occurred to him because of a medical tradition of using poisonous metallic elements as medicine antedating Galen and revived in the sixteenth century by the great German physician Theophrastus Bombastus von Hohenheim, who took the scientific name Philippus Aureolus Paracelsus. The problem was to find a dosage that would attack the disease and not kill the patient. When Cumming brought him a flybitten mare at Kolobeng, Livingstone gave it two grains of arsenic in a little barley daily for about a week. An eruption resembling smallpox broke out and forced him to stop the treatment. He tried the same dosage again later, but the mare refused the barley. Six months after exposure to the fly the mare died. Later, as we shall see, arsenical compounds became the major weapon against tsetse-borne diseases in man and animals.

The most troublesome disease on Livingstone's various expeditions was malaria. He was early sensitized to its dangers when his children came down with a dangerous fever on one expedition, and he himself suffered from malaria in 1853 and various times afterward. He observed on one expedition that "myriads of musquitoes showed, as probably they always do, the presence of malaria," but he did not connect the two more specifically.

He did use quinine to cure malaria with considerable success, however, and combined it with other substances in a pill. The bark of the cinchona tree of South America had been used to cure fevers around the world since the seventeenth century, but since malaria's fever and chills frequently strike again after an apparent cure its use had been controversial. Isolation in 1820 of the active ingredient, the alkaloid called quinine, made its manufacture possible and speeded its acceptance.

Livingstone used it to cure his children, and while exploring the Zambezi region from 1858 to 1860 his use of it enabled him to save all but three of his men—a remarkable feat in view of the losses suffered by Tuckey's and others' expeditions. His malarial pill, known to his associates as a "rouser," contained resin of jalap, calomel, quinine, and rhubarb. He allowed the first stage of rigor or chill to pass in malaria victims and waited for the second, the hot stage, to appear. When there was stoppage of secretion and headache, he then administered the pill and an hour later gave the patient five to ten grains of quinine. He continued the treatment every two or three hours until deafness, or cinchonism, set in. The greater the deafness, the more assured was Livingstone of his patient's ultimate recovery. For obstinate cases with prolonged vomiting and fever, the quinine treatment continued with the patient receiving five grains daily in his morning coffee.

Livingstone contracted malaria and survived it; he never contracted sleeping sickness, for neither the disease agents nor the appropriate species of fly lived in the area where he lingered longest. But with its effect on the animals he needed for transportation, the tsetse fly constituted one rugged cross among the many he had to bear in his explorations.

During David Livingstone's lifetime the white world's knowledge of Africa increased dramatically because so many travelers penetrated the continent. Their tales were avidly read, and the interest of governments, churches, and geographical societies was keenly aroused. Armed with quinine, explorers no longer faced mortal danger from every fever; greater perils now were the hostility of African kingdoms and the treachery of the Arabs and Africans who were bringing the slave trade in eastern Africa to its height of viciousness. Routes from the east coast to the fabulous lakes of East Africa became established, and the great controversy between John Speke, who discovered Lake Victoria in 1858 and asserted that it was the source of the

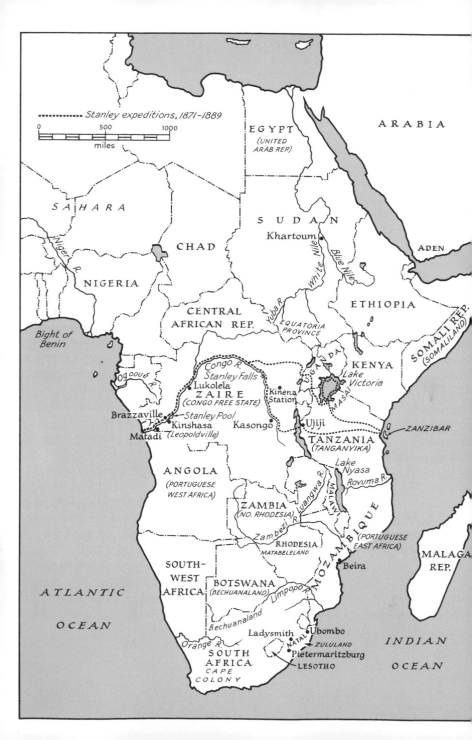

Stanley expeditions, 1871–1889

0   500   1000
miles

ARABIA

EGYPT
(UNITED ARAB REP.)

SAHARA

CHAD

SUDAN

Khartoum

ADEN

Niger R.

NIGERIA

CENTRAL AFRICAN REP.

White Nile

Blue Nile

ETHIOPIA

SOMALI REP. (SOMALILAND)

Bight of Benin

Juba R.

EQUATORIA PROVINCE

Ogooué R.

Congo R.
Stanley Falls

Lukolela

ZAIRE
(CONGO FREE STATE)

Kinena Station

UGANDA

KENYA
Lake Victoria

Brazzaville

Stanley Pool

Kinshasa
(Leopoldville)

Matadi

Kasongo

MASAI

Ujiji

ZANZIBAR

TANZANIA
(TANGANYIKA)

ANGOLA
(PORTUGUESE WEST AFRICA)

Lake Nyasa

Rovuma R.

ZAMBIA
(NO. RHODESIA)

Luangwa R.

MALAWI

Zambezi R.

MOZAMBIQUE
(PORTUGUESE EAST AFRICA)

MALAGA REP.

RHODESIA
MATABELELAND

Beira

SOUTH-WEST AFRICA

BOTSWANA
(BECHUANALAND)

Limpopo R.

ATLANTIC OCEAN

Bechuanaland

Orange R.

Ladysmith

Ubombo

NATAL

ZULULAND

INDIAN OCEAN

SOUTH AFRICA
CAPE COLONY

Pietermaritzburg

LESOTHO

Nile, and his rival, Richard Burton, who insisted Lake Tanganyika was the source, was finally resolved in Speke's favor.

Henry M. Stanley played the principal role in settling this controversy. An Englishman born in humble circumstances, he became a newspaperman and carved out a career as an enterprising reporter in the United States. His paper, the *New York Herald,* and the *Daily Telegraph* of London had financed the trip in 1871 to find David Livingstone, and his narrative of this encounter, *How I Found Livingstone,* inserted the phrase "Doctor Livingstone, I presume?" into the folklore of the English-speaking world. One passage of this book describes his encounter with the tsetse fly, called "chufwa" by his companions. He found it less formidable to man than two other types of flies which he examined when they invaded his tent, but it was most dangerous to animals. "Horses and donkeys streamed with blood, and reared and kicked through the pain," he wrote, perhaps exaggerating the case.

In 1874, Stanley's newspapers dispatched him to settle the Nile controversy, still raging ten years after Speke's death. He took with him a prefabricated boat which he assembled and launched on Lake Victoria, and he spent several months sailing round the shores of that great lake. Stanley thought that one or two rivers feeding into the lake might be the true source of the Nile, but British geographers declared in 1877 that the lake with their queen's name should bear that honor.

Stanley followed this feat by crossing central Africa from the east coast to the west, sending out exciting dispatches along the way. In the course of this journey he followed the Lualaba River; this turned out to be a tributary of the Congo which he then traced to its mouth. His letters also encouraged European leaders to think that penetration of the continent was not so difficult as it had seemed and aroused the interest of people who viewed the country he described as a field for commercial ex-

)f Africa showing Stanley's expeditions. (Drawn by John Morris.)

ploitation. This turn of events had profound consequences for the human disease transmitted by tsetse fly.

But Stanley's letters had another long-range effect. They helped to convince missionary doctors and other men to come to Uganda, men who would be of great service when epidemics later ravaged that kingdom. On the evening of April 14, 1875, writing from Usavara near Kampala, Stanley penned an appeal to be published in the *Daily Telegraph* and the *New York Herald* for a Christian mission to be sent to the court of Mtesa (the Measurer), the Kabaka or King of Buganda. The letter was a direct outgrowth of questions the Kabaka had put to him about religion. Stanley wrote:

It is not the mere preacher, however, that is wanted here. The bishops of Great Britain collected, with all the classic youth of Oxford and Cambridge, would effect nothing by mere talk with the intelligent people of Uganda. It is the practical Christian tutor, who can teach people how to become Christians, cure their diseases, construct dwellings, understand and exemplify agriculture, and turn his hand to anything, like a sailor—this is the man who is wanted. Such an one, if he can be found, would become the saviour of Africa.

Stanley's job description of 1875 for a missionary in Uganda reflected David Livingstone's pragmatic philosophy about missionary work—save the body as well as the soul. The immediate effect was to encourage a variety of missionary groups to establish operations in Uganda, each to woo the Baganda to its particular version of Christianity. The Muslims had a head start owing to the well-established Arabic trade and slave operations throughout East Africa. French and English, Catholic and Protestant missionaries quickly set up posts in Uganda. Within three years of Stanley's appeal, the Church Missionary Society of England had placed two of its missionaries in the country. In succeeding decades a series of minor religious wars broke out throughout the area, and many local Christian converts were persecuted. When for financial reasons the Imperial British East Africa Company had to abandon the area, the English missionary elements in combination with other interests in Uganda forced the British government to establish a protectorate over the territory.

The long-term impact of Stanley's letter was perhaps more beneficial, for it inspired young men to train for medical careers in Africa. We shall trace this effect in more detail below.

The news from Africa attracted the attention of young King Leopold II of the Belgians. In 1876 he created the International Association for the Exploration and Civilization of Africa. This association, organized on the advice of prominent ge ographers of those times, never functioned as an international institution, but it provided King Leopold with the initial administrative framework that led to the creation of the Congo Free State as his own personal domain, recognized as such in 1884.

In 1878, after having failed to interest the British government in the Congo, Stanley entered the service of Leopold to explore and develop the potential for commerce along that great river. Stanley spent the next four years in the Congo, paying special attention to that strip of river from its mouth at Matadi up the cataracts to Leopoldville (now called Kinshasa) and Stanley Pool. Nearly a century later in 1970, transfixed in stone, dressed in field clothes and tropical helmet, he stood in forward marching stance in the presidential gardens where the cataracts begin, overlooking the shipyards of Kinshasa close by and the twin cities of Kinshasa proper and Brazzaville on opposite banks of the pool upstream. In his service to Leopold he also pressed three hundred miles upstream to Lukolela and from there several hundred miles farther to Stanley Falls.

The French followed suit, for they, too, began to realize the richness of the natural resources of equatorial Africa, which the Congo River drained. On their behalf the Italian Pierre Savorgnan de Brazza explored what is now the Central African Republic and signed treaties with the African chiefs on the north banks of the Congo to bring their areas under French protection and domination.

In opening up the river to the modern commerce of that day, Stanley was instrumental in altering the riverine habitat in favor of that crocodile-loving, canoe-riding fly, *Glossina palpalis,* and he unwittingly became a harbinger of sickness and death. Up to this time sleeping sickness—still commonly known as Negro lethargy—apparently was limited to West Africa and the lower Congo. Thomas Winterbottom, a physician practicing in West Africa, had described in 1803 "a species of lethargy, which they are much afraid of, as it proves fatal in every instance." He had found this disease on the coast of the Bight of Benin. His description of the swelling of the neck glands as an early indication of the disease led this symptom to become known as "Winterbottom's sign." Robert Clarke reported his observations of the disease in Sierra Leone in 1840 and suggested that it was more common in the interior than on the coast. But signs of the disease's spread appeared with the quickening of commerce. A French naval surgeon, Armand Corré, wrote in 1876 that the *maladie du sommeil* had decimated several garrisons in lower Senegal and had caused some villages to be abandoned. Angola recorded its first case in 1871 and many more shortly after. The Portuguese government sent a scientific commission to investigate, but it made no real progress.

When Stanley arrived in the Congo, the riverside villages were small and isolated; the lines of communication tenuous. He put steamboats on the river, and the fly used them for passage. He detailed his men to build garrisons upstream, and the fly brought the disease into these growing population centers, which then served as foci for hinterland infections. His contact and that of his men with Arab slavers who had come to the Congo years before from the east coast stirred up *palpalis*. The famous—some would say notorious—Tippu Tib, of mixed Arabic and African blood, was one of these. The traders' movements about the heart of the continent facilitated the travel of this vector with its diseases eastward to the lake region of middle Africa.

Stanley's success in helping King Leopold to exploit the Congo triggered a whole chain of events which we now see disseminated the disease more rapidly and more effectively than ever before. King Leopold knew nothing about tsetse when, in 1876, he organized the African International Association (later Association Internationale du Congo), nor when this, his personal development agency, went far in transforming the Congo into a prosperous "Mississippi" river of commerce predisposed to the spread of flies and sickness—the river which Vachel Lindsay depicted thus:

> Then I saw the Congo, creeping through
>   the black,
> Cutting through the forest with a
>   golden track.

At that time no one, including Stanley and his lieutenant E. J. Glave, associated the tsetse fly with sleeping sickness, although Stanley, at least, felt it was a nuisance. This lack of knowledge, combined with Leopold's and Stanley's avarice in exploiting the Congo, helped permit epidemics of this disease to grow unchecked along the river.

E. J. Glave was a Yorkshire youth bent on adventure in Africa. At first he had difficulty in convincing the right people that they should employ him, but he peppered the African International Association with letters pleading that they accept him as a young recruit for Stanley's project on the Congo. Finally they did, and he soon earned his place as one of Stanley's pioneer officers. He arrived at Matadi in 1883 with three other Englishmen, and the four of them set out on the two-hundred-mile march along the Congo to Leopoldville, Stanley's headquarters. On the way, two of the Englishmen died of African fever (it could have been malaria); the third, broken in health, returned to England. Glave came through virtually unscathed, but he too must have contracted malarial fever, for Stanley commented that in Leopoldville Glave appeared gaunt, stooped, pallid, and generally sickly, while after several months upstream he emerged as the robust, healthy young officer he ought to have been.

After Glave had spent a month in Leopoldville, Stanley needed someone to build a station in the district of Lukolela, a compact, forested spot situated on the bank of the Congo about three hundred miles above Stanley Pool. He offered Glave the choice of this post or one in a place that was already cleared and had comfortable housing. Glave chose the dank jungle spot.

Later, in his 1893 book, *Six Years of Adventure in Congo-Land,* he described one incident that told better than do a thousand pages of documentary evidence about the fearsome contact the Congolese had with sleeping sickness there and, hence, with *G. palpalis.* Most of the 5,000 to 6,000 villagers of the Lukolela district near Glave's garrison knew about sleeping sickness. Glave strolled through one of their villages one day and found that they had dropped their tools and left their homes. Even a pot of "a fine savory stew of crocodile, monkey, and red peppers," as Glave put it, "resented the inattention paid to it" and had tipped over, putting out the fire. The people had congregated around two villagers who, armed with pangas, had slashed one another until each, standing in a pool of blood, was about to drop from exhaustion and admit he was beaten. The immediate cause of the fight: One had cursed the other, " 'Owa na ntolo' (May you die of sleeping sickness)."

Sleeping sickness, Glave explained, was a

mysterious disease peculiar to Africa, and incurable even by the cunning of their charm doctors. A native apparently in the best of health will be suddenly attacked by a continual desire to sleep, and within a very few weeks he will be so overcome by the malady that he will only wake up occasionally from sound sleep into a dreamy stupor, which period is occupied in the voracious consumption of food, and while thus engaged he will fall off again into his previous comatose state. One so afflicted rapidly wastes away to a mere skeleton, and then dies. . . . "Owa na ntolo" . . . is a direct challenge to fight, and no one but a coward will fail to accept it.

Both of the combatants survived, to Glave's amazement. They managed to walk to his garrison the following day, and with a varnish brush he applied carbolic oil as a salve to their wounds.

The hex in the invective "Owa na ntolo" had, of course, earned its spooky authority through past unfortunate experiences of many more than the two men who clashed at Lukolela. It portended disaster to large populations, not simply to a few individuals. The Irish "Traitor or Patriot?" Roger Casement, hanged in World War I for his activities as an Irish nationalist, found this out in a series of "tours" he made to Africa, tours which spanned twenty years.

Born in 1864 in Dublin, Roger Casement went to Liverpool in the mid-1880's to take up employment with the Elder Dempster Shipping Company. In 1884 he was able to satisfy his yen to travel to West Africa as a purser on one of the company's ships. Like Glave, he was fascinated by the continent and had an intense desire to return.

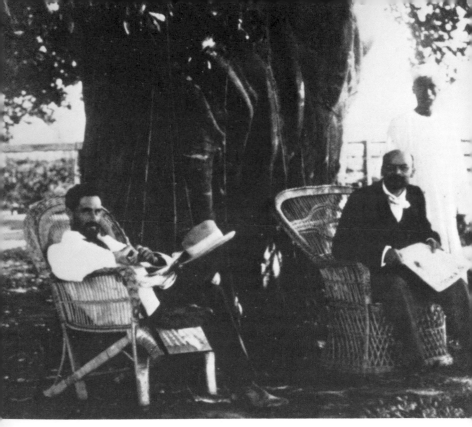

Roger Casement (*left*) in Africa. (Photograph from Herbert O. Mackey, *The Crime against Europe,* by permission of C. J. Fallon Ltd.)

Stanley was so famous that Casement could not aspire to join one of his expeditions. But in 1886 Henry Shelton Sanford was organizing an expedition. Sanford, an American tycoon and diplomat who had founded the town of Sanford, Florida, had secured United States recognition for King Leopold's African International Association before the Berlin Conference of 1884–1885, at which the European powers had divided Africa among themselves and recognized Leopold's claims. His objectives were to send forth explorers expressly to visit all villages along the banks of the Congo and its tributaries and to search for marketable products of the land. Casement became a part of this expedition, and Glave, on Stanley's advice, also joined it.

On this trip in 1887 Casement saw the Congo as a river with great potential whose exploitation the Belgians were conducting in a reasonable manner. On a subsequent lecture tour in the United States he said the Sanford mission had revealed the potential of Africa "for the benefit of the white peoples and for the *uplifting* of the Africans themselves" (italics added).

Later, Casement became involved in the development of another country, Nigeria, as Travelling Commissioner for the Colonial Office. While on that assignment he visited Sierra Leone and there recognized Winterbottom's sign. In 1892, Casement entered into correspondence with the famous British expert on tropical disease, Dr. Patrick Manson, concerning this symptom and the seriousness of the disease. Manson's biographers, his son-in-law, Philip H. Manson-Bahr, and A. Alcock, quoted and summarized Casement's comments about the enlarged lymphatic glands and the local treatment:

"The medicine man," wrote Casement, "after feeling the hard lumps embedded in the muscle round the back of the neck and in the glands of the throat, worked them up clear of the veins and then, with a rough country-made lancet, laid them open to view." A needle was passed through each lump and, the thread being drawn after it, a loop was formed and the hard white masses drawn out of the flesh and muscles. Five or six such operations were performed and the wounded parts wrapped up with a covering of leaves and palm-oil and bandaged to keep out the cold. Strong native purges were then administered during one or two days, to clear thoroughly all the impure matter out of the blood.

The treatment did nothing to cure the disease.

In 1900, after Colonial and Foreign Office assignments in Portuguese East and West Africa and in South Africa, Casement was sent back to the Congo—first to King Leopold's

Congo Free State, then in 1901 to Brazzaville in the French colony on the northern bank of the Congo. His reports to Whitehall confirmed earlier rumors of appalling labor conditions in the Congo Free State. Casement returned to King Leopold's Congo in June 1903 at the request of the British government to chronicle the labor relations between the Belgians and the Congolese. He gathered factual information on the conditions of forced labor and virtual slavery to which the Belgians were subjecting the Congolese, notably in the gathering of rubber. And he noted the growing incidence of sleeping sickness in the area.

Casement found the government stations in the Congo admirably built and well kept; he saw good business, a prosperous river, and fine lines of communication. But he also saw a diminished and an exhausted population. A fleet of steamers, forty-eight (he thought) in number and the property of the Congo State, navigated the main river and its principal tributaries at fixed intervals. Regular means of communication were available to some of the most inaccessible parts of Central Africa. An excellently constructed railroad over the difficult country which at an earlier date Glave and others had been able to travel only by foot connected Stanley Pool to the ocean ports. It was becoming easy for people, pests, and diseases to travel.

Leopoldville in those days consisted largely of a government station—which Casement likened to a barracks—of approximately one hundred and thirty Europeans and three thousand native workmen. There were also about twelve other Europeans and two hundred other Africans in Leopoldville. Here Casement inspected the two hospitals, one for Europeans and the other for Africans. The latter he characterized as "an unseemly place." It comprised three mud huts in dilapidated state, two with their thatched roofs almost gone. "Seventeen sleeping sickness patients, male and female," were "lying about in the utmost dirt," most of them on the bare ground. One woman had fallen into the fire just prior to his arrival. She was in the final, insensible state of the disease. Badly burned, she had been well bandaged but was still "on the ground with her head almost in the fire, and while [he] sought to speak to her, in turning, she upset a pot of scalding water over her shoulder."

On earlier visits Casement had found five thousand members of the Bateke tribe occupying three major towns near Stanley Pool, each within a few miles of the other. By 1903 there were only a few scattered European homes, and in Leopoldville just one hundred, perhaps, of the original natives or their descendants. Forced labor and virtual slavery conditions accounted in large part for the depopulation, but sleeping sickness was also a factor. Casement, viewing Stanley Pool and the cataract region of the Congo River below as the home or birthplace of sleeping sickness, termed it "a terrible disease, which is, all too rapidly, eating its way into the heart of Africa."

Upriver at Lukolela, the district that Glave knew so well and that he himself had visited in 1887, Casement met the Reverend John Whitehead, an American of the Baptist Missionary Society. He verified with his own eyes the state of that village as Whitehead had depicted it some months earlier, in July 1903, in a letter to the governor-general of Congo State:

The population in the villages of Lukolela in January 1891 must have been not less than 6,000 people, but when I counted the whole population in Lukolela at the end of December 1896 I found it to be only 719, and I estimated from the decrease, as far as we could count up the number of known deaths during the year, that at the same rate of decrease in ten years the people would be reduced to about 400, but judge of my heartache when on counting them all again on Friday and Saturday last to find only a population of 352 people, and the death-rate rapidly increasing. . . . The pressure under which they live at present is crushing them; the food which they sadly need themselves very often must, under penalty, be carried to the State post. . . . So far the officials of the State have never attempted even the feeblest effort to assist the natives of Lukolela to recover themselves or guard themselves in any way from disease.

Whitehead suggested that the small population of Lukolela be requested to vacate its present site and move to higher ground, that no one known to have "sleep-sickness" be permitted to dwell on the new site, that all be compelled to bury their dead at a considerable distance from their dwellings. To these he added many additional recommendations, most related to better sanitation, and none, significantly but naturally enough, to the expedient of controlling or eradicating *G. palpalis*. But then, at that time, neither he nor anyone else knew that this fly was transmitting the disease.

The outcry which resulted from Casement's 1904 report forced King Leopold to surrender his personal control of the Congo to the Belgian Parliament in 1908. But in spite of Leopold's harsh practices as an employer, he had attempted to attack the sleeping sickness in his colony. In 1903 he invited the Liverpool School of Tropical Medicine to send a team to the Congo to study the problem; Drs. J. Everett Dutton and John Todd set forth in September of that year and were soon joined by Dr. Cuthbert Christy. Dutton and Todd spent nearly a year and a half conducting investigations of sleeping sickness in the Congo, much of the time at a hospital which had been especially established for the purpose. Dutton died at Kasongo in February 1905 of tick-borne relapsing fever.

The writer Joseph Conrad, who hired out as a riverboat captain on the upper Congo in 1890, just for the experience, corroborated the stories of Glave, Casement, and Whitehead; he made the same journey on foot through the "Heart of Darkness" that they had made up the cataract region of the river to Leopoldville. Conrad met Casement and wrote of him, "A limpid personality. There is a touch of the conquistador in him too. . . . He could tell you things! Things I've tried to forget; things I never did know. He has had as many years of Africa as I had months—almost."

But Conrad "could tell you things" about the Congo and about sleeping sickness, too. He saw the railroad workers on forced assignments suffering at all stages of the disease. He wrote in *Heart of Darkness:*

Black shapes crouched, lay, sat between the trees leaning against the trunks, clinging to the earth, half coming out, half effaced within the dim light, in all the attitudes of pain, abandonment, and despair. . . . they were nothing earthly now—nothing but black shadows of disease and starvation, lying confusedly in the greenish gloom. Brought from all the recesses of the coast in all the legality of time contracts, lost in uncongenial surroundings, fed on unfamiliar food, they sickened, became inefficient, and were then allowed to crawl away and rest. These moribund shapes were free as air— and nearly as thin. I began to distinguish the gleam of the eyes under the trees. Then, glancing down, I saw a face near my hand. The black bones reclined at full length with one shoulder against the tree, and slowly the eyelids rose and the sunken eyes looked up at me, enormous and vacant, a kind of blind, white flicker in the depths of the orbs, which died out slowly. The man seemed young —almost a boy—but you know with them it's hard to tell. I found nothing else to do but to offer him one of my good Swede's ship's biscuits I had in my pocket. The fingers closed slowly on it and held—there was no other movement and no other glance.

Yes, *G. palpalis* with its deadly disease, taking advantage of those poor souls, was on the move.

The great lakes region of Africa experienced biological stresses and strains from exploration and development similar to those of the Congo basin. But in 1890 and 1891 when Emin

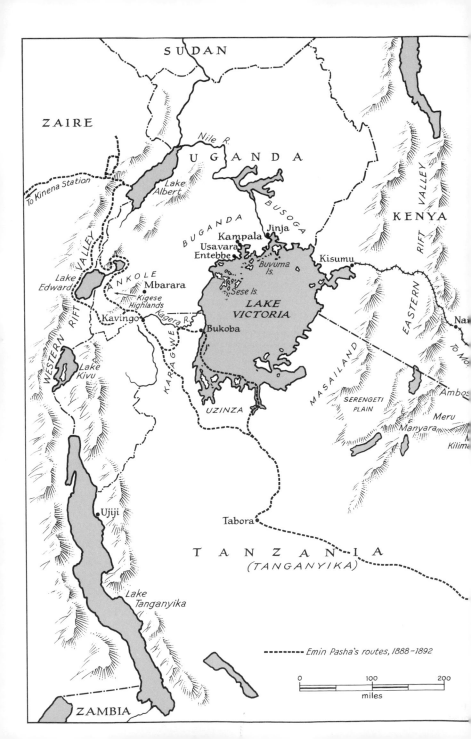

Pasha, his six European colleagues, and his retinue were exploring that region and built Bukoba as a German garrison on Lake Victoria, it seemed singularly unencumbered by the diseases *G. palpalis* and *G. morsitans* carried. *G. morsitans,* if present on cattle, was certainly quiescent along the shores of the lake and out to the hinterlands when Speke, Stanley, Lugard, Emin and others explored that highland area prior to 1900. *G. palpalis,* the man-biter, apparently had yet to infect people with sleeping sickness in noticeable numbers in this part of East Africa. These two insects surged into prominence in the wake of other scourges, including sand fleas, *Tunga penetrans,* and cattle plague.

Sand fleas probably entered the continent in West Africa in the 1870's or 1880's in sand ballast loaded in ships returning from Brazil, where they had delivered slaves. The fleas soon became established in the heart of Africa at Stanley Pool on the Congo. Like *G. palpalis,* they traveled quickly from there along the steamship route to Stanley Falls. By 1891 they had spread through the western branch of the Rift Valley to Livingstone's town, Ujiji, and over its eastern escarpment to Bukoba and Tabora.

The flea did not cause its damage by spreading disease. Female sand fleas buried themselves under the toenails of those who went barefoot and burrowed in other parts of the human body, too. When they became engorged with blood they created large sores which festered and became gangrenous.

Since most of those afflicted did not know what was causing their sores or at first understand how to cope with this problem, the flea debilitated the population in and about present-day Malawi, Tanzania, and Uganda. Robert Stephenson Smyth Baden-Powell—who would draw on his African experiences when he founded the Boy Scout movement years later—noted the movement of the sand flea during the British campaign to suppress

the Lake Victoria region of Africa showing Emin Pasha's routes. (Drawn by orris.)

the African uprising of 1896 in Matabeleland, now part of Rhodesia:

> We hear that the jigger, an insect the size of a pin's head, is invading South Africa. He came from the West Coast, and is now down as far as Beira. I know the beast: he got me coming back from Kumassi, and planted his eggs under my toe-nail, and I had ten minutes' genuine fun while the doctor cut them out.
> Curious how the little pest should be able to cross Africa, and make himself a scourge in a new bit of country,—just as the rinderpest has done,—taking three years to get here from Somaliland.

In Uzinza, an area along the south shore of Lake Victoria, one of Emin's German companions, Dr. Oscar Baumann, saw people with whole limbs rotted off as the result of sand flea attack. For want of laborers, fields went unharvested; entire villages died out.

All one had to do to combat sand fleas was to pick them out right after they burrowed into the flesh. But the local people had had no previous experience with this pest, so it took them time to realize how important it was to employ a technique so simple or, alternatively, to wear shoes if they could. The time it gained was just what the sand flea needed to work its damage.

Rinderpest, a virus disease of both domestic and wild animals spread not by an insect but through the air, entered the Busoga area from the east, also at the heels of Emin Pasha and other great explorers. The disease is highly contagious and nearly always fatal, characterized by inflammation of the respiratory passages, high fever, labored breathing, bloody mucous discharge, and leathery, diphtheria-like false membranes in the throat. It was therefore much more devastating than the sand fleas. It had periodically invaded Egypt but had not penetrated southward along the Nile to the lake region of East Africa until the epidemic of 1890, which Frederick Lugard and Emin Pasha witnessed.

Lugard, who in later years became one of Britain's best-known colonial administrators, was at that time a young professional soldier disappointed in love. He joined the Imperial British East Africa Company in 1889 and spent the next three years exploring and helping Britain solidify her claims to parts of East Africa. He blamed the cattle plague invasion of the 1890's on the importation of infected cattle from either Arabia or India to the east coast of Africa opposite Aden in 1889. He said that Italian armies advancing up the Blue Nile in Ethiopia carried the disease southward. Rinderpest reached Masailand and Uganda in 1890, and it spread south to Lake Nyasa in about July of 1892. Lugard wrote that "never before in the memory of man, or by the voice of tradition" had the cattle died in such numbers. These were areas where the livelihoods, the life styles, the very social orders of the people depended on cattle. The effect was devastating.

The area which received the full brunt of the sand flea and cattle plague invasion included Ankole, Karagwe, and part of Masailand, among other African political units. Ankole, in present-day Uganda, lies west of the shores of Lake Victoria where the Baganda people live. Like Karagwe and parts of Masailand, it is hilly range and grassland country. Today an arterial highway of asphalt running from Kampala on the lake west to the Ruwenzori Mountains, often called the Mountains of the Moon, cuts Ankole in two. Midway, the Agip Motel under the sign of the yellow dragon at Mbarara depends upon Ankole beef to serve its customers fondue Bourguignon and upon the fruits of the Kigese highlands to serve them strawberries with cream. Karagwe, in what is now Tanzania, is west of Lake Victoria, south of Ankole; it fans out on either side of the Kagera River, which flows east into the lake north of Bukoba. Masailand straddles Kenya and Tanzania southeast of Lake Victoria; it embraces what are now the Serengeti Plains, Manyara, Amboseli, and Meru game reserves.

The Bahima, a pastoral conquering tribe, dominated the old

Karagwe Kingdom. Their oral tradition plumbs nearly four hundred years of well-organized political and economic history back to about 1580. In the nineteenth century, these people, who derived their leadership from a type of inherited monarchy, lived in apparent harmony with the Banyambo of Karagwe, a peaceful, agricultural people whom they had subjugated in earlier days. John Speke and James Grant went "tripping down the greensward" of "this charming Land" in 1861 in the course of their attempt to discover the source of the Nile before Richard Burton did. Emin Pasha came through Karagwe with Stanley en route to the coast and recommended it to the Germans for development after he joined their command in 1890; he described it as an ideal area for cattle herding. He tarried there on his last expedition of 1891–1892 before he went on to Kinena Station in the Congo, where Arab slavers murdered him.

Karagwe territory did indeed support a thriving cattle industry. Local chieftains maintained standing herds of five hundred to a thousand long-horned, humpless cattle. To amass a "government" herd, the Germans under Emin employed techniques the local people also used but did not condone. They staged a series of forays, rustled cattle from their "rightful owners" and readily rounded up six hundred head.

In Karagwe Kingdom, the Bahima helplessly watched rinderpest nearly exterminate their stock—they lost 95 per cent of their wealth. Dr. Franz Stuhlmann, the zoologist of Emin Pasha's expedition into the interior for the German government, remarked on the large and well-cared-for herds they saw in Karagwe in March 1891. "Soon after our visit," he added, "a cattle sickness broke out, which brought all to the ground, so that the Bahima are now forced to engage in agriculture." W. Langheld, another of the party, observed the first attack early in 1891. The "government" herd of over six hundred head rapidly dropped to thirty-five. A period of recovery followed, but six months later the disease struck the thirty-five head that remained. It no longer mattered who rustled cattle from whom. At Kavingo, Chief Mukakikonjo presented Dr. Emin with several oxen, hoping that he in turn would supply him with medicine that would cure his cattle of rinderpest. Emin had nothing to offer and sent Mukakikonjo away, telling him that as a cattleman he should know how to control cattle plague better than Emin.

In Ankole, Chief Ntare would not see young Lugard. His cattle were dead, and he was ashamed to be visited in his poverty and starvation. He and his subjects were driven to eat what the local agriculturalists could provide and to try to follow their art of cultivation. Many people died, unable to produce food or to accommodate themselves to a vegetable diet. Those who did survive, Lugard wrote, were "thin and half starved, and much liable to a loathsome skin disease or 'itch.'" The malady was smallpox, which followed so quickly upon the rinderpest that many thought they were two forms of the same disease.

In Masailand, at least two-thirds of the whole Masai people were ruined. The warriors at first carried themselves through the disaster by hunting and petty thievery, but the women and children and old men, completely abandoned as they were to misery, "tottered through the steppe, feeding on honey of the wild bees and on nauseating carrion," as Dr. Baumann observed.

In Karagwe and Ankole, livestock maintenance and agriculture steadily deteriorated after the rinderpest outbreak. As the cattle disappeared, distasteful coarse grasses and thorn trees replaced the red oat grass, which the cattle loved. Bush crept over the cultivated fields and the pastures, creating an environment favorable to the tsetse fly. No longer could one see the extensive grazing lands which had supported large standing herds of cattle kept in previous years by people who loved them for the beauty and the grace of their horns rather than for the quality of their flesh.

Sometime during the last years of the nineteenth century, *G. morsitans* spread northward from the Rhodesias to this new hospitable environment in Karagwe. By 1909 *morsitans* had advanced at least seventy miles through the valleys of Karagwe to Ankole, and in 1947 a veterinary officer, John Ford, and a historian, R. de Z. Hall, could report Karagwe to be a waste of tsetse bush with small human populations crowded into congested hamlets as a defense against the spread of nagana on cattle. These densely populated hamlets were circumscribed with larger areas of cleared land than were individual households in the bush. These clearings acted as more effective barriers to the fly. Cattle kept in them away from the bush were less likely to be bitten by tsetse.

Karagwe Kingdom might have deteriorated anyway, for the Bahima were running out of strong and wise leadership by the 1880's and 1890's; but Emin Pasha and other great explorers certainly helped accelerate the disintegration of Karagwe and other chiefdoms.

Emin Pasha was one of those unusual individuals who qualified, in fact at times excelled, in the full range of categories listed in the daisy-petal-picking rhyme: "rich man, poor man, beggarman, thief; doctor, lawyer, merchant, chief." But his expertise as a scientist and his zeal for collecting natural history specimens knit his life and work into a consistent pattern.

Born Eduard Schnitzer of a protestant family in Silesia, Germany, in 1840, he earned his medical degree at the University of Berlin in 1864. He went to Turkey and there became attached to the staff of a prominent official, Hakki Pasha, as a tutor for his children. Hakki Pasha died in 1873 and Emin, who had fallen in love with Hakki Pasha's wife, acquired his widow and an instant family of eleven children. Two years later he abandoned this family, took the shortest route to Egypt, and entered the service of that government under the name Emin (the faithful one) Effendi. He professed the Moslem religion, but both his assumed name and his new religion seem to have been guises that enabled him to immerse himself thoroughly into the society of Egypt and the Sudan so as to be effective in his work as a doctor and a naturalist. Sociable, he was an accomplished pianist, good at chess, and a remarkable linguist.

From Egypt, Emin went to Khartoum, the capital of the Sudan, then to Equatoria, the southernmost province of that country where in 1878 he served as chief medical officer. General Charles (Chinese) Gordon, a Britisher, was at that time serving as an agent of the Egyptian government in Equatoria. In 1877, Gordon became governor-general of the Sudan and he appointed Emin as governor of Equatoria Province.

Emin's governorship of Equatoria extended over an eleven-year period, 1878–1889, when Egyptian influence in the Sudan was weakening. The Sudanese flocked to a local Moslem leader, the Mahdi, who repudiated Egyptian rule and its reliance upon Turks and other Europeans occupying high administrative posts. The Mahdists besieged and captured Khartoum, killed General Gordon, and effectively cut Emin's communications along the Nile. As the Mahdists advanced southward, Emin fled from Lado, the capital of Equatoria, and settled at Wadelai close to the mouth of Lake Albert with a remnant army of fifteen hundred together with their followers numbering close to ten thousand.The Mahdi never pursued Emin to Wadelai and he and his retinue eked out a hand-to-mouth existence there in isolation for seven years.

Emin's whereabouts and plight concerned leaders in Europe and provided Stanley with the excuse for an expedition, highly publicized, to come to his rescue in 1888. For months after

Stanley found Emin, they wandered together around Lake Albert and in Equatoria Province until Emin finally made up his mind to accompany Stanley at least to the East African coast, where they arrived with a collective force of nearly six thousand followers. Here at Bagamoyo, near Dar es Salaam, at a celebration of the "success" of the expedition, Emin suffered a serious accident. His vision impaired by cataracts and used to living in one-story houses, he walked by mistake over the edge of a second-story balcony and fell eighteen feet to the ground; he broke several ribs and fractured his skull.

As Emin recuperated he decided against returning to Europe as Stanley's exhibit of a model rescued explorer. He turned to the German government, which financed his last exploration to the Lake Victoria region, to assist that government to establish and strengthen its claims as a colonial power in East Africa. This trip, in company with Langheld, Baumann and Stuhlman, took him into Masailand, Ankole, and Karagwe. From there he traveled without his companions to Kinena station in the Congo, where he was murdered.

In 1891, on this his last expedition, at fifty-one, nearly blind, still collecting birds, methodically recording his observations, beset by hostile Africans, Arabs, and mutinous colleagues, Emin asked himself in a moment of despair: "Why is it that I alone, among all those I knew, am still a rolling stone?" Emin's personal motives and professional rationalization—to do anything as long as what he did gave him freedom to pursue his scientific interests—accounted in part for his wandering in Africa. But part of the answer to his question surely lay beyond his control, in the nature of man as an incorrigible carrier and disseminator of his own diseases and of those of his livestock. Like Stanley, Emin was a mover of people and he stirred things up.

On his trips through East Africa hundreds of men formed

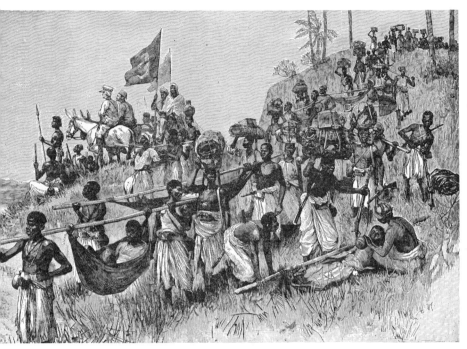

Emin Pasha, Stanley, and their "army" marching to the coast. (Engraving, The Bettmann Archive.)

part of Emin's expeditions. When he made his trip to the coast in company with Stanley, many of them stayed in the lake region of East Africa. Some of these men were infected with sand fleas, and these people served as a source of infection for others who did not yet have them. They and newly infected people became debilitated and less able to cope with other diseases such as smallpox and syphilis, which had become rampant.

The livestock Emin and his men herded no doubt came in contact with livestock infected with rinderpest, contracted the disease, and then transmitted it to uninfected herds. In killing cattle, rinderpest prepared the land for bush encroachment and the advent of tsetse.

In East and Central Africa, foci of rinderpest remained; it became endemic in these areas and periodically seeded new outbreaks. From Karagwe, Ankole, and Masailand, rinderpest stormed south through the Rift Valley. In a matter of months it reached what is now the Republic of South Africa. On the way it cleaned out buffalo, waterbuck, reedbuck, warthog, and bushpig. It also took eland, sable, wildebeest, giraffe, and many other species of wildlife.

As rinderpest swept through what is now Rhodesia, the measures undertaken by the government (Cecil Rhodes's British South Africa Company) included the slaughtering of sound cattle. Baden-Powell reported in his book on the 1896 uprising of the Matabele that these people thought this was part of a European plot to destroy them and added it to their list of grievances against the British.

When rinderpest advanced south of the Limpopo River in April 1896, the Cape Colony government, one of the precursors of the Republic of South Africa, made a desperate effort to protect its extensive cattle herds from this plague. It constructed a barbed-wire fence just south of the Orange River from the border of Bechuanaland with southwest Africa, southeast to present-day Lesotho, then along the Cape-Natal border to the Indian Ocean, a distance of more than a thousand miles. Mounted police patrolled the fence, and the government depopulated a wide neutral zone of all susceptible animals along the border. Clothes of European travelers moving south were disinfected; the entrance of Africans was practically prohibited.

The disease broke through in 1897 despite all precautions.

Authorities traced the penetration to the leader of a span of trek oxen who had picked up a sack of dried meat, presumably infected, and who had donned a pair of blood-stained trousers he had found nearby. His oxen, in contact with him, contracted the disease. As they moved down one of the main roads, they passed it along to others south of the border, who spread it further until rinderpest had killed more than 2,500,000 head of cattle in South Africa alone. The speed and thoroughness of its attack held one blessing; it killed susceptible species so completely that no lasting source of infection remained for subsequent infestation.

But the Cape Colony government had taken other measures to combat rinderpest. In 1896 they had called Robert Koch to South Africa and he began to immunize cattle in a crude but scientifically accurate manner. He relied on what cattle herders had already observed—that the bile of infected cattle had disease-inhibiting properties. He slashed the dewlaps of healthy cattle and inoculated them with bile from infected ones. This method supplied uninfected animals with the antibodies to combat the disease and was practical to use. By the end of 1898 rinderpest was under control in South Africa.

The immediate effect of rinderpest on tsetse is disputed. Some said the losses starved the fly out for lack of wild and domesticated stock on which to feed. Others felt that tsetse simply became more vicious and turned in greater numbers to man and to the few animals which were left for food.

In 1900, less than ten years after rinderpest on cattle spent itself in eastern Africa, Congo-born *Glossina palpalis* and sleeping sickness possessed the shores of the greatest of all African lakes, placid Victoria. Livingstone and Emin Pasha, who had roamed Eastern Africa, were dead. Stanley lived in virtual retirement in Britain. Roger Casement had yet to make his second trip up the Congo. The Boer War had broken out in South Africa, and an army doctor named David Bruce had been recalled into regular army service to take charge of a military hospital in Ladysmith during the siege of that town. The Imperial British East Africa Company had nearly completed the construction of the railroad from Mombasa to Kampala, and the company had turned over governing British East Africa to the Foreign Office of the British government. The Foreign Office had set up two protectorates—one for Uganda, the other for Kenya. Tanganyika, now Tanzania, was in the hands of the Germans.

At this time, Lake Victoria, almost the size of Lake Superior, was truly an international waterway—far more than today when jet airliners pass over it carrying passengers scarcely aware of the lake below. Steamboats used it to connect Kisumu on the Kenya shore with Entebbe on the Uganda side. Missionaries, doctors, and government servants used them. Canoe traffic was also heavy, especially to the islands in the lake. Half-sunken hippopotami, like massive boulders come to life when disturbed, harried pilots and paddlers seeking haven. The crested crane, Uganda's national bird, occupied the shore lines while other birds controlled the lake's flyways or fished in it for the tasty *Tilapia*.

No one worried about *G. palpalis*. In 1900 no one yet knew that tsetse carried sleeping sickness. But sleeping sickness would cast a pall over Kampala (the home of the impala) and over other towns in Buganda along the lake—the area Winston Churchill labeled a "curious garden of sunshine and deadly nightshade."

During the first decade of the twentieth century the tsetse fly began to depopulate parts of Uganda—the population of the Buvuma group of islands, on the Equator in Lake Victoria, dropped from 56,000 people in 1900 to 13,000 in 1907. The Busoga area, on the north shore of the lake east of Buganda, was as badly affected. Busoga, known by some as a prosperous banana garden area, become notorious for epidemics of smallpox, syphilis, and plague, for famine, and for political upheaval. To determine the severity of the sleeping sickness epidemic here, the government instructed the local chiefs to report to headquarters and to carry with them a twig to represent the death of each individual they thought died of sleeping sickness within their chiefdoms. A solemn procession of chiefs came to headquarters on the first day and the twigs numbered eleven thousand. The chiefs continued to bring bundles of twigs to headquarters for several days afterward.

Hospital facilities were completely inadequate to receive the vast number of patients suffering from a disease which no one had the slightest clue how to cure. Moreover, the local people customarily handled the problem by abandoning the victims. Uganda's Principal Medical Officer, Dr. R. U. Moffat, who was grandson to the earlier Robert Moffat and nephew to David Livingstone, wanted to set up a sleeping sickness concentration camp on Buvu Island to isolate the victims of the disease. But Buvu was not a good choice, for it was heavily infested with biting flies—tsetse, of course—which would have transmitted the disease even more rapidly. Poised to set up the camp, he received cabled instructions from Britain to abandon the project; the Royal Society would send out a commission instead. The population along the narrow band of fertile lakeshore of Uganda which *G. palpalis* occupied dwindled from 300,000 to 100,000, and the country as a whole lost a tenth of its people to sleeping sickness.

The epidemic that crippled the population of Uganda probably had been incubating for a quarter of a century. This span of time, 1875 to 1900, almost coincided with that of Henry M. Stanley's working years. When Stanley crashed through the jungle from the Congo to Uganda to rescue Emin Pasha, sleeping sickness carried by *G. palpalis* must have followed him. The people of Uganda would not know this until years later because those species of tsetse already there had been biting them for centuries and never seemed to do them any harm.

The nineteenth century had thus wrought fundamental changes on the African continent south of the Sahara. Its isolation from the rest of the world and the isolation of its regions from one another were ended. First the Arabs and Portuguese, bent on trade in ivory and men, had penetrated the unknown interior, then came other western Europeans searching for geographical knowledge, opportunities for commerce and colonization, and souls for Christ. Transportation routes were established, many served by railroads and steamships, and European powers had carved up the continent for development and exploitation. The centuries-old slave trade, which had reached its peak of cruelty in East Africa, had been abolished, but new forms of control were imposed on more people, some in ways that could hardly be distinguished from slavery. Moreover, European development had unwittingly made it possible for native and imported diseases to ravage human populations and their animals. Thus European influence, in large part intended to do the African people good, presented on its other face a curse. Now it was the time for other Europeans, with their own ways of thinking and methods of organizing, to seek the formulas to ease the curse.

Asking the Right Questions

*I have not the slightest belief in the notion popularly prevalent up
to the present that the Fly causes the disease by the injection of a
poison elaborated by itself, after the manner of the leech, which in-
jects a fluid to prevent the coagulation of the blood, or the snake
for the purpose of procuring its prey or for defence, but that at
most the Tsetse acts as a carrier of a living virus, an infinitely small
parasite, from one animal to another, which entering into the blood
stream of the animal bitten or pricked, there propagates and so
gives rise to the disease*

David Bruce
*Preliminary Report on the Tsetse
Fly Disease or Nagana, in Zululand*

In 1894 the British army posted one of its career doctors,
David Bruce, in South Africa for ordinary duty. When he arrived at Pietermaritzburg, Sir Walter Hely-Hutchinson, a distinguished Knight of Ireland who had been lieutenant governor of
Malta when Bruce had discovered the cause of undulant fever
there, was serving as governor of Zululand and Natal. Sir Walter realized that fly disease was destroying an alarming number
of cattle in Zululand and believed that Bruce should be assigned the task of determining its cause and cure. Through his
influence, Bruce was seconded from military duties to work on
59   this project.

Bruce at the time was thirty-nine years old. He had been born in Australia but had been raised from the age of five in Stirling, Scotland. Though he left school at fourteen to start a career in business, his interest in natural history led him to enter Edinburgh University at the age of twenty-one to study zoology. Soon he switched to medicine, was graduated in 1881, and worked for a time as an assistant to a physician.

He entered the army medical service and was stationed in Malta from 1884 to 1889, where he demonstrated his skill in finding the causes of disease. When he arrived on the Mediterranean island, the British garrison was hospitalizing six hundred to seven hundred men a year for an average of 120 days each for what was called Malta fever (undulant fever). Bruce studied all aspects of the disease. In 1886, following the bacteriological approach of Karl Joseph Eberth, Edwin Klebs, and Robert Koch, who in the early 1880's had discovered the organisms causing typhoid fever, diphtheria, and tuberculosis, Bruce found and identified a bacterium (*Micrococcus melitensis*) in the spleens of men who had died of the fever; he demonstrated that it caused the illness. This bacterium was later named *Brucella* in his honor, and Malta or undulant fever is now known also as brucellosis.

On his first leave in 1888, Bruce and his wife, a doctor's daughter who worked as his laboratory assistant and illustrated his scientific papers, stayed with Koch in Germany and studied his bacteriological methods. Koch himself spent some time in South Africa, where he developed a vaccination technique to combat rinderpest, as described earlier.

From 1889 to 1894, Bruce was on the faculty of the Army Medical School at Netley, England. Then he received his orders for South Africa and his assignment to study the tsetse fly disease. Late in December 1895, he submitted to Hely-Hutchinson a twenty-eight-page report describing the work he had done, the

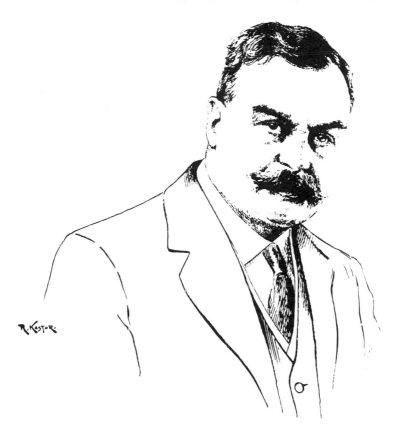

David Bruce, March 31, 1925. Bruce inscribed the picture "Nil sine magno—Vita labore dedit mortalibus." (Sketch, The Bettmann Archive.)

results obtained, and his conclusions. This, subsequently published as *Preliminary Report on the Tsetse Fly Disease or Nagana, in Zululand,* became one of the classics of parasitology. "Nagana" was a Zulu word meaning low or depressed in spirits;

Bruce's use of it established it in the English language. He could have used "munca," which the Zulus also used; it describes the "sucked out" appearance of affected animals.

As one would expect, a report of this sort did not include certain details about Bruce's experiences. We learn from other sources of his earlier association with Hely-Hutchinson, and of his first contacts with the disease and with the tsetse fly itself in Pietermaritzburg. The report does not tell of the early experiments he performed by crushing flies in alcohol and inoculating animals with the macerated mess to see whether the flies carried some poison as a snake does. It skips the Bruces' first journey by oxcart to Ubombo in Zululand and their labor to convert a two-room hut with a grass roof, which belonged to an early settler married to a Zulu, into laboratory and living quarters. And it does not dwell on the frustrations which tenuous communications brought on; Bruce was recalled to Pietermaritzburg in 1895 for what proved to be no good reason, and the unnecessary trip caused a seven-month pause in his nagana experiments, though he used the occasion to study another cattle disease, red water fever. The report presents in a clear, logical fashion the facts he found to answer questions he posed.

According to this document, he investigated three hypotheses. One was the view, which he attributed to Europeans, that the bite of "the Fly" caused the animals to sicken and die. Another was the belief, which he said was held by many Africans in Zululand, that large game contaminated the grass or drinking water by their saliva or excretions and that this brought on nagana. The third attributed the disease to tropical conditions in general and more immediately either to malaria or to a vegetable poison.

The evidence he marshaled began with an attempt to infect an "English" dog with flies that had not been exposed to the disease (dogs had long been known to be highly vulnerable to nagana). He carefully shaved the dog's abdomen and let five flies feed there for more than two months. The dog remained perfectly healthy. Next he exposed a "native" dog to the bites of flies that had previously fed on a dog known to have nagana. This dog developed the illness. These tests showed that the fly itself did not cause nagana but readily carried it from affected to healthy animals. Perhaps Bruce, knowing that his hypothesis was strong, instinctively gave the English dog, presumably the more highly prized, the exposure that led to negative results.

Bruce next tried to determine whether the fly transmitted the disease in nature. He repeated Vardon's experiment of fifty years earlier, taking horses into fly-infested country and allowing them to be bitten, to see if they would come down with the disease. Three healthy horses, muzzled while in fly territory so they could not contract nagana from something they ate or drank while there, subsequently developed nagana. This result was not decisive, Bruce pointed out; the disease could have come from something the horses had breathed in. But he continued: "For my part I have much difficulty in believing that animals are infected as a rule with Fly Disease by inhaling the materies morbi, and until I find animals still susceptible to the disease which are protected in some way or other both from feeding and the fly, I shall continue to be sceptical."

To close the case and prove that tsetse was transmitting nagana in nature, Bruce began to bring flies up daily from the fly country to feed on susceptible animals. In a rather breathless postscript to the report dated six days after the report's submission to Hely-Hutchinson on December 12, 1895, he said that a healthy horse so exposed unquestionably had contracted the disease. Therefore, he concluded, "I consider myself justified in believing that the Tsetse Fly in a state of nature does convey the disease to susceptible animals."

Even more important than his establishing the fly's role in transmission of nagana, however, was Bruce's discovery of the organism that caused it. He had found the culprit by examining the blood of infected animals under a microscope with a magnification of five hundred. He wrote:

The Red Blood Corpuscles are seen as small faintly yellow discs, and among them and causing much commotion among them, can be seen transparent elongated bodies in active movement, wriggling about like tiny snakes and swimming from corpuscle to corpuscle, which they seem to seize upon and worry. They appear to be about a quarter of the diameter of a Red Blood Corpuscle in thickness, and 2 or 3 times the diameter of a corpuscle in length. They are pointed or somewhat blunt at one end, and the other extremity is seen to be prolonged into a very fine lash, which is in constant whip-like motion. Running along the cyclindrical body between the two extremities can be seen a transparent delicate longitudinal membrane or fin which is also constantly in wave-like motion.

Bruce cautiously called the creature only "the Haematozoon or Blood Parasite of Fly Disease." But he added, "in all probability on further knowledge it will be found to be identical with the haematozoon of Surra, which is called Trypanosoma Evansi or at least a species belonging to that genus." His second guess was correct. The parasite was a new species of trypanosome, a protozoan microorganism assigned to the animal kingdom rather than the vegetable, to which bacteria belong. The species has been named *Trypanosoma brucei,* or Bruce's trypanosome.

Trypanosoma means "auger-body." The parasite received this name because it frequently moves about in spiral motion like an auger bit. In 1843, Gruby of Paris had given the name to the species he discovered in a frog. The first known identification of a trypanosome occurred in 1841, when a Doctor Valentine of Berne saw one in a trout. The first observation of trypanosomes in the blood of a mammal was made by Timothy

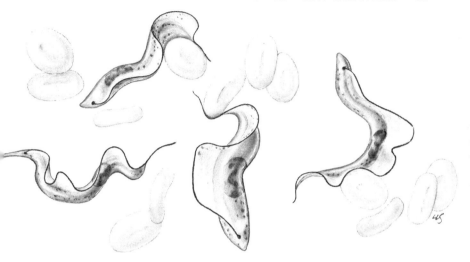

Trypanosomes amid red blood corpuscles of animal blood (Drawn by Lonna Lagreco Scott.)

Lewis in 1878 in rats in India; this species became known as *T. lewisi*. In 1880, Griffith Evans saw trypanosomes in the blood of horses and camels suffering from a disease called surra in India, and this type was named *T. evansi*.

Merely finding an organism in a sick animal is by no means proof in itself that the organism caused the disease. Microorganisms are often found in a perfectly healthy man or animal, and an innocent microorganism may be found in one sick with a disease caused by something else. Such circumstances had long confused the search for causes of other diseases—malaria, for example—and would enormously complicate the investigation of sleeping sickness during the first decade of the twentieth century. Following Koch's bacteriological methodology, however, Bruce established that his trypanosome caused nagana with the following chain of evidence:

1. It is found in the blood of every animal suffering from this disease, and is absent from the blood of all healthy horses, cattle or dogs.

2. The onset of the disease is marked by a rise in temperature, and this corresponds with the first appearance of the haematozoa in the blood.

3. As the disease progresses, pari passu [at equal pace] with the destruction of the Red Blood Corpuscles the parasites tend to become more numerous, sometimes reaching the enormous number of 5, 10, or 15 millions in every drop of blood.

4. The transference of the smallest quantity of blood from an affected to a healthy animal sets up the disease in the latter, as I have shown above, even the very small quantity of blood conveyed by the proboscis of a few Tsetse Flies is sufficient to carry the disease from animal to animal.

This evidence naturally disposed of the hypothesis that nagana was caused by malaria or a vegetable poison.

As Livingstone had before him, Bruce experimented with arsenic to try to kill the trypanosomes in the blood of horses. While Livingstone's dosage had been two grains daily, Bruce gave one of his horses twelve grains. He used two separate dosages a day, each containing six grains of arsenic and six grains of carbonate of soda in an ounce of water. He scattered the fluid over the horse's grain, adding sugar after the horse seemed to develop a distaste for the arsenic and grain alone. Under this treatment the horse regained its strength and for nearly two months carried him down to fly country and back every other day when he went to collect flies. Eventually it also died, as did the other horses both treated and untreated in the series of experiments.

Bruce did not trace the life cycle of the trypanosome. It was later shown that trypanosomes pass through an eighteen- to twenty-four-day stage of development in the fly, during which time they cannot transmit the disease. For laboratory transmissions men can force immediate "mechanical" passage of uncycled and still virulent trypanosomes from one host to another, but this is difficult and the usual method is to rear a clean fly, let it feed on an infected animal, wait until the fly becomes infective, then have it feed on an uninfected animal.

He did, however, add entomology to his accomplishments by studying the life cycle of the dark-eyed, smoky-winged tsetse that was causing nagana in Zululand. Like all species of tsetse, it laid no eggs but instead extruded, one might say gave birth to, a yellow larva nearly as large as the ringed, pale yellow abdomen of its mother. The larva was legless, looking rather like a plump worm, was divided by rings into ten segments, and had a black hood at one end and two minute spikes at the other. Immediately after birth it energetically crept around in search of cover. Having found a suitable resting place, it gradually changed from yellow to jet black and from a soft, wiggly form to a hard, rigid pupal case. At this point Bruce left the experiment because he had to return to Pietermaritzburg, but he had left some pupal cases under leaves, others under moist earth, and still others in dry places, and he was confident that at least some would produce a new generation of adult flies ready to take up trypanosomes from infected animals and pass them along to others. Later, in his *Further Report,* he noted that the life cycle had progressed as he had expected.

The preliminary report and its less famous successors constitute an epochal chapter in the story of an able man who started out as a doctor, and, responding to the force of circumstances, became an outstanding bacteriologist, then turned protozoologist, and finally excelled as an entomologist. His role in our story is by no means ended.

But Bruce was not dealing, as he thought, with Cumming's omnipresent *Glossina morsitans.* His description of his specimen approximates the one that Major Austen published for

G. pallidipes (pale-footed tongue-fly). "Legs buff-coloured; middle tarsi, like the front pair, entirely pale." These are the distinguishing marks of *G. pallidipes*. It had been identified as a species a few years earlier from specimens collected far away in East Africa.

Bruce, concerned with its role in the transmission of nagana, worked at the southernmost tip of its range. At its northernmost limit, near the slopes of Mount Kilimanjaro, the British had been racing the Germans to complete a railroad from the coast inland. The collectors here were Frederick J. Jackson, later deputy commissioner for the Imperial British East Africa Company in Uganda, and Richard Crawshay, working on the Uganda Railway. With four thousand Indian laborers to manage and the competition to worry about, other problems far outweighed that of the fly. To them it represented only a nuisance, judging from a note by one—"settled on back of collector's neck and bit him." Yet they took the trouble to send flies to E. E. Austen at the British Museum in London while Bruce at the time did not, and so they went down in history as collectors of the type specimens.

The spread of sleeping sickness soon gave cause for concern that the fly was far more than a mere nuisance. As the toll of sleeping sickness grew, doctors and scientists in Europe and Africa turned the techniques developed in bacteriology and parasitology toward the search for its cause. Two of these were brothers, Albert and Jack Cook, both missionary doctors in Uganda. Their presence there was due in part to Stanley.

The Cooks grew up in a family where the pressures to study medicine must have been strong. Their father was a well-to-do doctor, and their older brother became a practicing physician in Britain. Sometime during his early years Albert read Stanley's famous appeal for practical missionaries for Uganda, which had been published when he was five years old. Added to the influences immediately around him, the letter must have encouraged him to switch his studies from the arts, in which he had begun, to the sciences, in which he clearly excelled.

Shortly before he qualified for his medical degree, Albert Cook also heard Stanley give an address on Uganda as he received an honorary doctorate from Cambridge University. Again Stanley told of the need for medical missionaries. In 1896, Albert left for that land to build a hospital and to practice medicine in Kampala under the auspices of the Church Missionary Society. Four years later his younger brother, Jack, fresh from medical school, joined him.

Powerful personalities who in time towered over their contemporaries as missionary doctors, the Cooks were also superb clinicians wedded to their microscopes. Imagine Albert's exasperation when, on the arrival of his party in Mombasa, the porters banged about the case containing his delicate microscope, perhaps the first in Uganda. Government doctors fared just as badly; they had to haggle with balky customs officials who insisted that microscopes fell into the high-duty category of musical instruments.

The Cooks arrived at the time when sleeping sickness was apparently still unknown in Uganda. On February 13, 1901, "Dr. Jack" consulted his brother about two patients in their hospital who appeared to be suffering from sleeping sickness. These evidently were the first hospitalized cases in the epidemic that was to ravage the population along the shores of Lake Victoria. "Dr. Albert" took blood samples from the patients, examined them under a microscope, and found filariae, threadworms about four times longer than the diameter of a red corpuscle, swarming in both. The brothers also found filariae in three of their next five sleeping sickness cases, and they notified the government.

They also informed Dr. Patrick Manson, the English physician with whom Roger Casement had corresponded, who was well known for his work with similar threadworms. In 1879, early in his extremely successful and colorful career in the Far East, Manson established the fact that the mosquito acts as an intermediate host for *Filaria bancrofti,* the worm that causes the extreme enlargement of limbs known as elephantiasis. Having amassed a considerable fortune in Chinese dollars, he returned to England in 1889 to retire. But the Chinese dollar underwent a devaluation and retirement became difficult. And so, fortunately for medical science, he returned to work, this time as a physician at the Seaman's Hospital in Greenwich. He was appointed medical consultant to the Colonial Office in 1897 and later served the Foreign Office in a similar capacity. He became widely known as "Mosquito Manson," partly because of his work on elephantiasis but more because of his persistent defense of the theory that his colleague Ronald Ross advanced and in 1898 demonstrated to be correct—that mosquitoes transmit malaria.

"Guided by the divining-rod of a preconceived idea"—in this case the wrong one—Manson overrated the importance of threadworms as causal agents of disease. He conjectured that a species *Filaria perstans,* now called *Acanthocheilonema perstans,* similar to the one he knew in China, might cause sleeping sickness. As evidence he could point to its prevalence in the blood of the few sleeping sickness patients being treated in London by 1890. He recorded this notion in several works, including his influential manual *Tropical Diseases* of 1898, which was the Cook brothers' medical Bible in their sixty-six-bed hospital in Kampala. The Cooks' evidence strengthened Manson's hypothesis. But he was too good a scientist to proclaim on this evidence alone that the *Filaria* actually caused the disease.

Dr. Jack Cook published a widely read paper on sleeping

sickness in the *Journal of Tropical Medicine* for July 15, 1901; for this Manson contributed a foreword pointing out that a unique opportunity existed in East Africa to determine whether *Filaria* really caused the disease. With anxiety quickening as the number of patients with *Filaria* became known and as the sleeping sickness epidemic worsened, Manson was able to persuade authorities to form a commission to study sleeping sickness in Uganda. In 1902 he was instrumental in organizing such a group under the auspices of the Foreign Office and the Royal Society.

Two members of the first sleeping sickness commission— Manson's commission—came from the London School of Tropical Medicine, which Patrick Manson had helped found in 1899. One was Dr. George Carmichael Low, a bright man of thirty, understood to be, though not named as, chairman of the commission. As a threadworm specilist he was supposed to prove or disprove Manson's hypothesis that *Filaria persians* caused the disease. He later became superintendent of the school.

The commission's senior member was thirty-nine-year-old Dr. Cuthbert Christy, epidemiologist and member of the Royal Society. One reason for his selection was his experience in Nigeria. While Low had worked abroad in the West Indies and British Guiana, Africa was new to him, and the commission's sponsors thought he needed someone familiar with the continent to accompany him. Christy was upset at not having been designated chairman of the commission. When he arrived at Mombasa he was not on speaking terms with Low. It is reported that the two actually came to blows over the fact that at Mombasa their railroad compartment was reserved in the name of "Low and party."

The third member was the brilliant Aldo Castellani, an Italian hereditary count who was twenty-five years old and a stu-

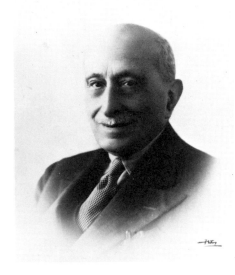

Count Aldo Castellani of Chisimajo, M.D., F.R.C.P. (London), F.A.C.P. (U.S.), President International Society of Tropical Dermatology, Membre d'Honneur Societé Française de Dermatologie, Fellow American Academy of Dermatology, Professor in the Institute for Tropical Medicine, Lisbon. (Courtesy of Frederick Reiss, M.D.)

dent of Manson's at the London school. A senior bacteriologist had first agreed to go, but at the last moment he decided to stay home, because his wife had just had a baby. In response to this emergency, Manson canvased his class in bacteriology for a replacement. All the students volunteered, and Castellani seemed best qualified. Before coming to London he had worked in the laboratory of Professor Walther Kruse, a famous bacteriologist at the University of Bonn. After the appropriate interviews at the Royal Society and the Foreign Office he was appointed the team's bacteriologist.

Castellani recalled in his memoirs that the next few days were spent gathering laboratory equipment together. Two days before the departure date, Low asked him, "What about your tropical outfit? . . . Do you expect to march into tropical Africa in a frock-coat?" Castellani described his shopping experience:

I . . . rushed to the tropical outfitters and bought two khaki suits, and was greatly attracted by a gigantic sun-hat of a most peculiar shape. It was a real monstrosity, with a large flattened dome and a huge peak in front, and attached at the back to the enormous brim, like a tail, was a long, broad red ribbon intended to protect the spine from the ultra-violet rays of the sun. My two colleagues never allowed me to wear that monumental headgear— they asserted it would make me and the whole Commission the laughing stock of Equatorial Africa.

That universal question, "What should I wear?" did make a difference in tsetse land. Even the donkeys wore clothing in the days of Castellani. The practical caravan leader traveling through the tsetse fly belts would frequently dress the donkeys in long trousers made of "Americana cloth" (cotton), which gave them a ridiculous appearance but protected them to some extent from fly bites. Some donkeys that were bitten became "salted," which meant that they had come down with nagana, recovered, and thereafter seemed to possess a degree of tolerance to the disease.

When the tsetse flies mobbed Albert Schweitzer and his paddlers as they were canoeing down the Ogooué River in the early 1900's, Schweitzer noticed that the flies pestered those among the party wearing white much less than those wearing other colors. In later years Kingsway, the supermarket chain in English-speaking Africa, sold an outfit consisting of a white open-necked short-sleeved shirt, white shorts, and knee-length white socks. Except for the exposed areas, one is reasonably well protected by this clothing because it is white. At the "sundowners," or cocktail hours, heavy white socks seem safer and more comfortable than black ones on two counts. Before dusk tsetse flies will go to the black; after sundown mosquitoes are less likely to cluster around one's ankles.

Suitably equipped with tropical garb, Low, Christy, and Castellani arrived in Mombasa in June 1902 and set out for Uganda. On the way they visited the Reverend Dr. C. A. Wiggins, Medical Officer at Kisumu, Kenya. "A queer lot," Wiggins termed them in his memoirs. "I've often wondered how such Commissions are chosen." An appropriate question to ask of commissions being formed even today.

In Uganda the members naturally met hostility and suspicion. The local doctors quite rightly thought that they might have more to contribute to the search for the disease's cause than the visitors had. Certainly they were working hard enough on the problem. The Cook brothers were frantically searching among the drugs available to them for some sort of effective medicament. The Principal Medical Officer of Uganda, Dr. R. U. Moffat, Livingstone's nephew, was trying to organize an isolation camp for sleeping sickness patients. Dr. C. J. Baker, employed locally by the Uganda government in Entebbe, was also struggling to combat the disease.

After much wrangling and hard work, too, the commission did not discover the cause of sleeping sickness. They had followed the wrong hypothesis. Thirty-five per cent of the sleeping sickness victims harbored no *Filaria perstans,* and 35 per cent of the people who did had no sleeping sickness symptoms. Christy, the epidemiologist, who had not accompanied his colleagues to Entebbe but had gone from Kisumu to Busoga where the sickness was worst, tried to match the geographical distribution of people with the parasite with that of people with sleeping sickness. Instead he found, as Wiggins had suggested from his own observations, that the little worm was found in a much wider area than the disease. Even today it has not been proved that the worm can be blamed for any human or animal malady.

The commission failed to develop another hypothesis, and in a few months Low returned to England. Christy, with some valuable maps of sleeping sickness to his credit, lost interest in the assignment after the *Filaria* hypothesis collapsed, and he spent most of his time hunting, collecting, and sending natural history specimens back home. He returned soon after Low and joined a commission of the Liverpool School of Tropical Medicine dealing with sleeping sickness in the Congo. Years later, on a hunting safari in the Congo, a rhinoceros turned on him and killed him.

But Castellani stayed on. Continuing his search for microorganisms in patients, he came across a *Streptococcus* bacterium in the blood and spinal fluid, grew it in a laboratory culture, and announced early in 1903 that "I think I have good reason to consider [it] to be the cause of sleeping sickness." Soon after he entered a dispute with a Portuguese commission investigating sleeping sickness in Portugal's African possessions over whether his bacterium was the same as one the Portuguese had already discovered.

Earlier, in November 1902, Castellani, using a new centrifuging method, had also found "a little fish-like parasite darting about" in the cerebrospinal fluid taken from the lower spinal cord of several patients. He recognized it as a trypanosome similar to David Bruce's but did not identify it as the cause of sleeping sickness at that time. But this discovery fitted other evidence and lines of thought that had been developing in recent years and also demanded investigation.

Bruce's work with nagana and the discovery of other trypanosomes in other animals has already been described. The credit for the first observation of trypanosomes in a human goes to a French physician, Gustave Nepveu. In 1891 he reported that he had seen them while looking for malaria parasites in the blood of a man in Algeria. But the significance of the finding was not noticed. In 1898 another Frenchman, Dr. Julien C. Brault, conjectured that trypanosomes might cause sleeping sickness. But he offered no convincing evidence, and no one paid any attention to this hunch.

A year earlier Patrick Manson missed a chance to link a trypanosome with a human disease. Examining under a microscope fresh blood from a patient in London, he saw a tadpolelike object swim across his field of vision. Then it was gone. So was the patient, who had left the house where Manson made the blood smear. Manson eagerly traced the man to his club, but by this time the patient was feeling the effects of his drinks and grew so belligerent that Manson had to give up trying to obtain further specimens of his blood. The episode was not described till much later.

The definitive link of a trypanosome to a disease of man was made in 1901. Robert Michael Forde, a surgeon serving as superintendent of a hospital at Bathurst, Gambia, in West Africa, examined the blood of an English steamship captain who was suffering from an irregular chronic fever. Through his microscope Forde saw a very active organism he could not identify. Dr. J. Everett Dutton of the Liverpool School of Tropical Medicine was present in consultation at a second examination and immediately identified the organism as a trypanosome. He named the parasite *Trypanosoma gambiense,* or Gambian auger-body, for the country in which it had been discovered, and the disease was called Gambian river fever, trypanosoma fever, or trypanosomiasis. *T. gambiense* was the organism Castellani also found two months after a description of the case was published.

Another physician, Alexander Maxwell-Adams, had attended the steamship captain's case. In March 1903 he published a note on trypanosomiasis suggesting that the disease took two forms—one in which the parasite circulated freely in the blood, when its symptoms were the chronic, irregular ones of trypanosomiasis, and another in which it accumulated in brain tissue, causing the lethargy and loss of function characteristic of sleeping sickness.

Finally, as a second sleeping sickness commission from the Royal Society was nearing East Africa in March 1903 to join Castellani, C. J. Baker, the obscure government doctor in Uganda, reported finding trypanosomes in the blood of an African policeman suffering from headache and fever. Baker diagnosed the case as trypanosoma fever. The discovery may have led him to wonder whether a tsetse fly, which he believed was unknown in the area, could be the vector as it was with nagana in animals. He may have had a role in launching a campaign to collect specimens of biting flies, for in a May medical journal he reported having been brought a tsetse. He and others apparently were unaware of the specimens Jackson and Crawshay had already collected in the area, a description of which Austen was preparing to publish in London.

Thus there was evidence that trypanosomes were present both in the blood of trypanosomiasis patients and in the spinal fluid of sleeping sickness victims, a suspicion that the disease could be borne by a tsetse, and the supposition that two apparently unrelated diseases were different stages of the same affliction. Clearly, then, this was a major direction of attack. All the pieces of a puzzle now lay face up on the table. It remained to be seen whether they fit into a picture. Almost by accident, the new commission's head was the best qualified man to find out whether they did—David Bruce.

The task of selecting the second commission's members had fallen to E. Ray Lankester, director of natural history of the British Museum, vice president of the Royal Society, and chairman of its Tsetse Fly Subcommittee, which had been set up following Bruce's discoveries in South Africa. "Big and bulky with rather a humorous face," Sir Hesketh Bell, governor of Uganda, wrote of Lankester. "I am told that he can be very rude at times." An inspiring and brilliant teacher and a notable scientist, Lankester had clashed with Manson several times in the past. He maintained, for example, that mosquitoes did not play an important part in transmitting the filariae of elephantiasis. Moreover, as a zoologist he equated tropical medicine with parasitology, a branch of biology best reserved to biologists. Medical men, he thought, were inadequately trained and therefore should stay out of it. But at this time he was unaware of Castellani's discovery and he had no reason to suspect that sleeping sickness was a parasitic disease.

At first Lankester recommended that Dr. David Nabarro, an 1898 graduate in medicine, head the new commission. Nabarro was a "small, quiet, rather mild and retiring man," according to an analysis of the commission's work by J. N. P. Davies, "but he was a determined man, a born scientist and his small frame covered a large heart. He was above all a man of courage and a fighter for causes in which he believed." But advisers warned Lankester that Nabarro could not get along with Castellani, who the society hoped would stay on. Nabarro wisely suggested that the society appoint an older man as the group's head under whom both he and Castellani could work.

Lankester, who was partial to the group of army specialists and doctors whose teaching and research operations were based at Netley, then recommended that Bruce head the commission. Bruce, after solving the nagana puzzle, had been recalled to more primary military medical tasks by the outbreak of the Boer War, and he had served as a surgeon in several battles and a siege. He had returned to England in 1901 to present the report of a committee to investigate enteric fever and dysentery in the army in South Africa. By the time of his appointment he was a lieutenant colonel and a fellow of the Royal Society.

The government approved his appointment on the commission—not, as it should have, because of Bruce's brilliant work with fly and trypanosome in Zululand, but because he was available and because he would cost it no more money, since he was already on the army payroll. The government had already refused to pay for the services of another senior scientist for the commission. Mrs. Bruce and a medical corps technician were the other commission members.

The combination of Bruce, Nabarro, and Castellani was certainly as bizarre as that of the first commission. Bruce was a forty-seven-year-old Scot, an intolerant Protestant at the peak of his career; Nabarro was a young, retiring Jew; Castellani a brilliant, ambitious Italian Catholic.

Castellani was suffering from a case of jangled nerves. His teammates had gone home, leaving him alone, and neither the doctors in Uganda nor the members of the Royal Society in London had warmed to his suggestion that the streptococcus bacterium he had found might cause sleeping sickness. On hearing of Bruce's appointment he foresaw problems in working under this eminent but reputedly arrogant man. He therefore agreed to stay only a few weeks after Bruce's arrival to demonstrate how he was obtaining specimens of spinal fluid and searching for microorganisms in them.

Bruce and his commission arrived in Africa on March 16, 1903, and Bruce departed August 28 the same year. In that brief time the commission had marshaled the evidence that proved that sleeping sickness was caused by a trypanosome carried by a tsetse fly.

In a report covering the work up to the time of his departure, Bruce built the case on the observation of trypanosomes

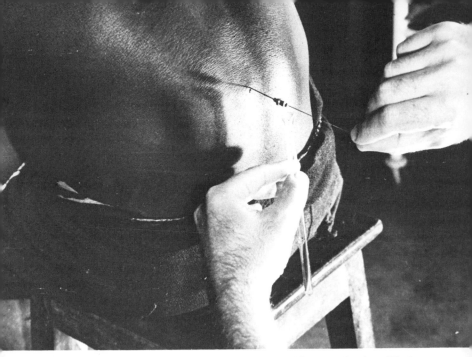

A lumbar puncture to collect cerebrospinal fluid for examination. (Photograph by N. B. Mitchell from 1966 *Annual Report,* by permission of the Nigerian Institute for Trypanosomiasis Research.)

in the blood and spinal fluid of sleeping sickness patients. When first detected by Castellani, the trypanosome could not be found in a high percentage of the cases, and the evidence seemed no stronger than for the disproved *Filaria perstans* or Castellani's bacterium. But improved examining methods revealed the parasite in the spinal fluid of all. Moreover, they were found by Wiggins in all cases in Kisumu, where patients had not harbored the *perstans* organism, and they were not found in the spinal fluid of people without sleeping sickness symptoms. In practically all cases trypanosomes were found in patients' blood as well.

Bruce then asked whether there was a relationship between trypanosoma fever and sleeping sickness, citing the case diagnosed by Baker and the descriptions from the west coast. The trypanosomes involved in both diseases appeared to be identical. Two of Baker's patients seemed to be passing on into sleeping sickness. Trypanosomes taken from a sleeping sickness case and from a man showing none of the symptoms both produced spinal trypanosomes and death in monkeys. "The evidence is not strong enough at present to justify a dogmatic answer to the question," Bruce concluded, "but what there is points to the trypanosomes being one and the same, and trypanosoma fever the first stage of sleeping sickness."

A comparison of blood samples inside and outside the sleeping sickness area was then reported. Eighty people from all over Uganda temporarily quartered in Entebbe to work off their "hut tax" were tested; twenty-three were found to have the parasite. An examination of fifty people in Nairobi, Kenya, which was free of the disease, turned up not one trypanosome.

The commission then turned to the tsetse and found that the *Glossina palpalis* species, first discovered in the Congo, was abundant in Entebbe's botanical gardens. The African prime minister and regents of Uganda were shown the fly. They immediately identified it as "kivu" and said it was found along the shores of Lake Victoria. A large-scale collecting campaign was then organized, and in three months the commission acquired 460 collections of flies and made a spot map of tsetse locations. Tsetse distribution coincided with the incidence of sleeping sickness plotted on a second map the commission drew.

Tests with the fly itself showed that it could transmit trypanosomes from an infected monkey to a healthy one if the second feeding came within forty-eight hours of the first. Flies collected in the hut-tax laborers' quarters were allowed to feed on healthy monkeys and transmitted trypanosomes to them.

On the basis of this evidence, Bruce concluded:

1. That sleeping sickness is caused by the entrance into the blood and cerebro-spinal fluid of a species of trypanosome.

2. That this species is probably that discovered by Forde and described by Dutton from the West Coast of Africa, and called by him trypanosoma gambiense.

3. That the so-called cases of trypanosoma fever described from the West Coast may be, and probably are, cases of sleeping sickness in the earliest stages. . . .

6. That the trypanosomes are transmitted from the sick to the healthy by a species of tsetse fly, *Glossina palpalis*, and by it alone.

7. That the distribution of sleeping sickness and *Glossina palpalis* correspond.

8. That sleeping sickness is, in short, a human tsetse-fly disease.

Though the previous false trails led some specialists, such as Manson, to treat the findings with caution, these conclusions were widely accepted. Indeed, earlier news had already prepared the ground. Castellani had left the commission and reported his discovery of the trypanosome orally to the Royal Society on May 14, 1903, and an account was published May 23, along with a summary of a telegram from Bruce of April 28. A German publication published a similar account May 18 based on information Castellani had given his former mentor, Walther Kruse, before reaching England. This note called the organism *Trypanosome castellanii,* or Castellani's trypanosome. Baker's report, published May 30, indicted the tsetse fly and said of a specimen that had been brought to him: "Colonel Bruce has assured me [it] is undoubtedly of the tsetse fly group, and he has kindly forwarded specimens to the British Museum for further identification." Lankester, in a preface dated May 15 to Austen's monograph on the tsetse, stressed the significance of Castellani's report and the importance it gave to knowledge of the fly. Christy, at a symposium on July 28, showed that his map of sleeping sickness incidence agreed with the reported habitat of *G. palpalis*.

Naturally the matter arose as to who should get what credit

for his contributions toward explaining the cause of a disease so important and complicated. Parties formed to stress the role of Bruce or Castellani and minimize the importance of the other, and an acrimonious conflict burst forth. In the abundant literature that followed, H. Harold Scott, in his *A History of Tropical Medicine* (1939), gave Castellani credit for the discovery and Bruce credit for recognizing its importance. Davies' analysis of the controversy stressed the underplayed contributions of Nabarro and Baker.

The description of the dispute needs no more detail here. Suffice it to say that the struggle for personal glory tested the integrity and eroded the reputations of both Bruce and Castellani and disturbed Nabarro greatly. Nearly sixty years later the last two, the only surviving members of the sleeping sickness commissions, said that their roles in discovering what causes and transmits sleeping sickness—one of the most significant discoveries in parasitology—had poisoned their lives.

Following their assignment in Uganda, the members of the team went their separate ways. Nabarro returned to England and became occupied with a variety of responsibilities in the field of pathology until he died in 1958. Castellani went to Colombo, Ceylon, as director of the tropical disease clinic. After World War I, he directed the Ross Institute of Tropical Medicine in London and later established the School of Tropical Medicine at Tulane University. In retirement he lived at Estoril in Portugal and died at the age of ninety-seven in 1970. Bruce took up where he left off in the study of Malta fever. As leader of the Royal Society's commission from 1904 to 1906 he spent part of each year with Lady Bruce in Malta, where he traced the origin of infection of Malta fever to the milk of Maltese goats. As luck would have it, further investigations of sleeping sickness were in the offing for Bruce. In 1908 he returned to Uganda with a team of technicians and stayed for two years. In

1912 he led a sleeping sickness commission to Malawi (Nyasa-land), where he worked out the relationships among the various species of trypanosomes infecting man, livestock, and wild animals. He died in 1931. An unsung later member of the Bruce, Nabarro, Castellani commission, Lieutenant Forbes Tulloch of the army medical service, became a casualty of the cause. He cut himself by accident while examining an infected rat. Evidently Tulloch himself became infected from the rat's blood, and he died of sleeping sickness in England a few months after his return there.

The cause of sleeping sickness was found, the way it infected people known. There remained to find a way to cure it. The fascinating story of how effective drugs were developed is told in detail later. At this point, arsenic and mixtures and compounds of that element seemed most worth trying. Bruce had treated horses in Zululand with arsenic and soda. His results had been mixed; some horses died, others seemed to become cured, still others got better and then suffered relapses.

Albert and Jack Cook, although their work was set back when their hospital, struck by lightning, burned to the ground, tried a variety of drugs. Sir Albert recalled after he had been knighted for the accomplishments of his career in Uganda that he once tried on forty-five people a "remedy put on the market by a firm of high reputation. . . . Every one promptly died." Prior to the availability of atoxyl the Cooks depended on intramuscular injections of "Liquor Arsenicalis," arsenious oxide.

One patient Sir Albert remembered was a young Ugandan whose cervical gland juice was

swarming with trypanosomes. . . . [I] gave him a series of injections of Liquor Arsenicalis, increasing very gradually until he received the equivalent of the truly astonishing dose of one and a half grains of arsenious oxide at a single injection. All symptoms disappeared, and a year and a half later he wished to marry. I examined his gland juice, and found a single living trypanosome. Treatment was recommenced, and he was allowed to marry. He was certainly alive twenty years later, for he used to send a modest thankoffering of two rupees to the Church annually.

The Germans in 1906 dispatched a sleeping sickness commission to their East African possessions. One of its members was Robert Koch, then sixty-four, widely regarded as the father of bacteriology. He settled on a fly-infested island in Lake Victoria about thirty miles from Entebbe and built a reed hospital there. Koch depended on another derivative of arsenic, atoxyl, which had been found effective against trypanosomiasis in animals. Atoxyl had also been used in Germany to treat anemia and skin diseases; it is sodium B-aminophenylarsonate, which has the staggering formula $NH_2C_6H_4AsO(OH)ONa$. This, like other arsenicals caused people pain and held a danger of damaging them physically, but no better drug was then in sight.

Koch started with half a gram of atoxyl in a single injection. Five days afterward he could still find trypanosomes in patients who received this dosage. He then doubled the dosage by administering half a gram on two consecutive days. This dosage kept the blood free of parasites for a long time, but to obtain even better results he stepped up the treatment to one gram about every seventh day for an indefinite period. Many patients could not stand the pain and absconded. Moreover, quite to the surprise of Koch and his associates, more than twenty patients who survived became blind. Such heavy doses of arsenic had damaged the optic nerve. The treatment was then reduced to half a gram every tenth day, which, while not perfectly effective against trypanosomes, was low enough not to cause blindness. This became the standard treatment.

While chemists and doctors were pressing their urgent search for drugs that would cure sleeping sickness in man, other scientists were vigorously studying the suddenly important tsetse and the microscopic protozoan it carried. An enormous aid was *A Monograph of the Tsetse-Flies* published by E. E. Austen of the British Museum in 1903, when the tsetse's chief economic importance seemed to arise from its role in spreading nagana and its similar relationship to human disease was just coming under suspicion. Austen had entered the British Museum in 1889. His first expedition took him to South America, where he served as naturalist for a voyage of the Siemens' Brothers Cable S.S. *Faraday* to the Amazon. Three years later, at age thirty-two, he turned his attention toward Africa on an expedition under the leadership of Major Ronald Ross which the Liverpool School of Tropical Medicine sent to Sierra Leone in 1899 to study the causes of malaria. There he collected *Glossina palpalis,* in fact was frequently bitten by this fly. A year later Austen was in South Africa, where he served the British army with distinction in the Boer War.

From his African experience Austen cultivated a lasting interest in flies, particularly the tsetse flies. He foresaw their potential significance, should they be discovered to be the vectors of sleeping sickness; he anticipated that doctors and others working in Africa would want to know everything there was to know about tsetse; and he hoped also to encourage all who would to send tsetse flies to him at the British Museum.

Austen's monograph listed only seven species; fifty years of subsequent studies by a number of entomologists have expanded that number to twenty-two. In Austen's day flies were flies, in the sense that even specialists had trouble differentiating one closely related species from another. The same still holds true, and most casual observers do well barely to recognize tsetse if, in fact, they can distinguish it at all from other biting flies. In setting forth a description, perhaps it is not possible to imprint clearly with words the image of a certain spe-

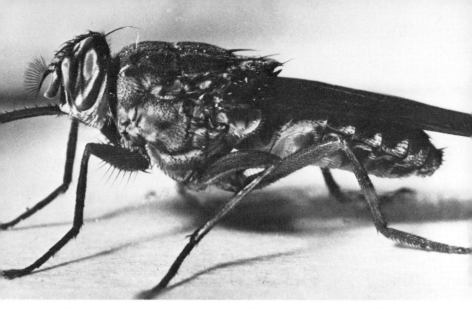

Adult tsetse showing its proboscis. (Courtesy of M. A. Prentice.)

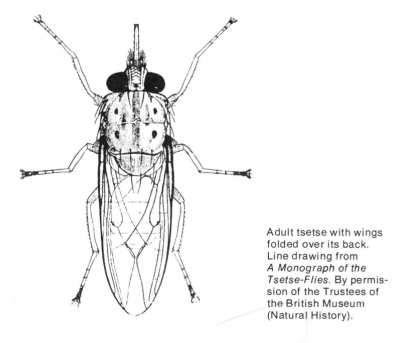

Adult tsetse with wings folded over its back. Line drawing from *A Monograph of the Tsetse-Flies.* By permission of the Trustees of the British Museum (Natural History).

cies of fly upon the mind of one who has never seen such a fly. Can one adequately describe a rose to another person who has neither seen nor smelled one?

Major Austen admitted that probably only those who had been bitten by tsetse would recognize it later "on the wing." But he pointed out, as have others before and after him, that identification of tsetse is easy when the fly is at rest. Their "brownish *wings lie closed flat over one another down the back,* like the blades of a pair of scissors, while *the proboscis . . . projects horizontally in front of the head."* Apart from these two characteristics there is nothing remarkable or striking about these ordinary-looking flies.

But the life cycle of tsetse is quite remarkable, as discovered by Colonel Bruce and as described many years later by Bernhard and Michael Grzimek in their book *Serengeti Shall Not Die* (1961). They pointed out:

Many people do not know that a fly can be pregnant. Ordinary flies, and most other insects, lay large numbers of eggs which hatch out into larvae. Most of these die. The tsetse fly has a different method. After the male and female have paired, which may take up to five hours, the female is fertilised for the rest of her life. If a fertilised fly should stray into a region where there are no others she will still continue to produce fertile eggs for the remaining two hundred days of her life.

She produces eggs but does not lay them. A female tsetse fly will hatch out a single egg inside her own body and feed the larva through special glands, similar in function to the uterus in mammals. The young larva will then shed its skin three times inside the "womb" just as ordinary insect larvae do outside the bodies of their mothers. Then the single larva is born as a whitish maggot, two-fifths of an inch long.

During the last few days before the birth the mother can no longer suck blood because there simply is no room for a meal. She chooses shady, loose soil as a nursery and uses her own legs to act

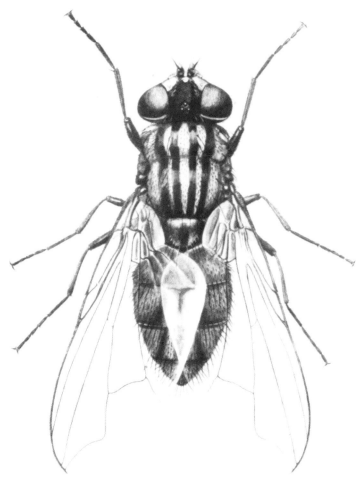

Adult housefly. (Drawing from Austen from Thomsen, from John Smart, *A Handbook for the Identification of Insects of Medical Importance,* 2d ed., 1948. By permission of the Trustees of the British Museum (Natural History)

as midwife. The larva burrows from sight within twenty minutes. Once inside the ground the skin of the larva hardens into a brown pupa, and within thirty-five days the maggot inside the chrysalis changes into an adult fly. When it is ready, the young fly opens the chrysalis by pushing at the lid with its head. It even has a special blister on its forehead specifically for this purpose. Once the young fly is free the blister disappears, probably because the air inside it helps to inflate the crumpled new wings. A fertilised female can bear two or three children a month.

Tsetse flies classify conveniently into three main categories; the first of these, the *G. fusca* group, includes twelve large dark species that average in size almost the length of the printed words "tsetse fly," about 12 mm. They live in the dense forest, rarely attack man, but pose a potential threat to cattle in those areas.

The second, the *G. palpalis* group, embraces five species, if one includes *G. fuscipes* as a species. Three of the five, *palpalis, tachinoides,* and *fuscipes,* constitute the main carriers of sleeping sickness. Small to medium-sized insects—a little longer than the word "tsetse," of about 9 mm.—they inhabit forest and riverine areas but they also reach out to some extent into the savannas of Africa.

The species of the third, the *G. morsitans* group, constitute insects of size similar to those in the *palpalis* group; they thrive in game areas. While three species in this group, *morsitans, pallidipes,* and *swynnertoni,* are the main carriers of nagana to cattle, two of them, *morsitans* and *swynnertoni,* especially, transmit the virulent Rhodesian strain of sleeping sickness to man.

At the turn of the century the curious person looked for size and color differences in the adult, in order to try to determine which species he had in hand. To arrive at a more precise identification he also had to count the bristles on its face and the hairs on its feelers; to check the color of its "feet," and to consider the places where it lived.

None of these characteristics was so striking as to absolve one from looking at tsetse ever more critically. Color of the five segments of the "feet," called tarsi, would help most to separate *G. palpalis* and *tachinoides* from *morsitans, pallidipes,* and *swynnertoni.* If one were to kill *palpalis* or to look at pinned specimens of this species with stretched-out wings, he would see a distinct light isosceles triangle on the back of the first segment of the abdomen, a marking that *tachinoides* does not possess. In *morsitans,* the most widespread species of the lot, only the last two of the five segments in the front and middle tarsi are dark, while in *pallidipes,* as its name would suggest, all five joints of the front and middle tarsi are light. *Swynnertoni's* main distinguishing features when it is compared with *morsitans* seem to be its large size and its black bands on a brown abdomen. Rare is the person, however, who will wait long enough to count the tarsal joints, let alone check their color, while tsetse pumps blood from his system.

If one turns a tsetse upside down, it is easy to tell the fly's sex because the male possesses a prominent "button" that the female lacks on the final segment of the abdomen. In the decades that followed the publication of Austen's monograph, entomologists came to use the reproductive organs of tsetse as ever more precise means for telling the species apart. In 1924, Professor Robert Newstead of the Liverpool School of Tropical Medicine built his revision of the genus *Glossina* on just such characters. Later, certain species were crossbred. If fertile progeny resulted, the two so-called species did not stand as truly distinct species. The twenty-two species accepted as valid today have undergone such tests of modern science.

To be able to identify a particular tsetse species accurately, a novice should frequent the places where they live and have a

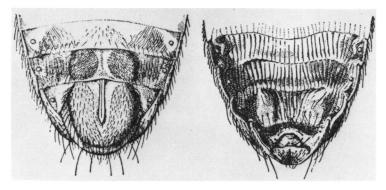

Underside of the tips of the abdomen of male (*left*) and female (*right*) adult tsetse flies. The male has a knoblike structure called hypopygium which is absent in the female. Drawing from John Smart, *A Handbook for the Identification of Insects of Medical Importance*, 2d ed., 1948. By permission of the Trustees of the British Museum (Natural History.)

specialist familiar with them point out the dominant fly in that region together with its companions. The Lake Manyara National Park in Tanzania affords him not only a good look at the fly but also a chance to feel its bite and maybe to catch sleeping sickness while he watches the herds of elephants and other big game.

Within the broad ecological bands outlined above, each species has unique "furniture requirements"—need for shade, logs, tree trunks, appropriate soil and debris conditions which fit that fly for comfortable living in certain types of bush or jungle country. *G. palpalis,* for example, normally follows the river courses, where it bears a major responsibility for transmitting the widespread Gambian trypanosomes causing sleeping sickness in people; sometimes it will desert shade entirely to investigate a possible food host. Occasionally it will even fly to a maize or millet field, or along the borders of cassava and cotton fields. It may rest for short periods on completely exposed

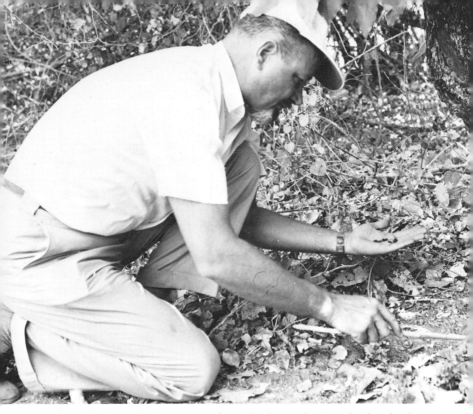

Investigator collecting pupae from the base of a tree in the riverine habitat of *Glossina palpalis* and *G. tachinoides*. (Photograph, United States Agency for International Development, 1964.)

rocks. On dull, cool days it may languish; during hot, thundery, or stormy weather and on dry bright sunny days it may become quite active.

Bright moving objects excite the interest of *G. palpalis*. Hungry individuals seem to be attracted to gray stones—probably instinctively, for close to them may lurk its food hosts such as crocodiles, lizards, hippos, and bucks. Like its distant relative, the housefly, *G. palpalis* shows a curiosity for almost anything new, but the curiosity subsides as familiarity with the object grows.

G. palpalis makes use of occasional trees and of bush along the rivers for breeding. Frequently a pregnant female alights a few inches from the ground on the underside of a stone, a fallen log, or, often, of an overhanging tree trunk or of any other object forming a small angle with the surface of the soil where she will drop her young. Larvae and pupae of tsetse may be found in large numbers under thick layers of fallen fig leaves.

G. tachinoides, the companion species of *palpalis* in West Africa, is a nervous, flitty fly better able to withstand heat and dryness. It reaches beyond and supplements the range of *palpalis* along the intermittent rivers, dry except in the rainy season, of the derived savanna zone of West Africa which, but for the cultivation and pastoral activity of people over the last several centuries, would today be forested. *Palpalis* has another companion in East Africa, in the Sudan, and in parts of Zaire—*G. fuscipes,* which for years was considered only a subspecies of *palpalis.*

G. morsitans, one of the most effective species in spreading trypanosomiasis on cattle, is not a riverine species; it occupies savanna-type areas instead. Its two "alter egos," *G. pallidipes* and *G. swynnertoni,* are somewhat fussier than *morsitans* about where they will live and consequently are restricted in range. *Pallidipes* claims as its home Natal, Zululand, and certain parts of East Africa; *swynnertoni,* named for Charles Francis Massy Swynnerton, one of the truly great naturalists of Africa, is limited to the big game country of East Africa, where some of the finest research ever in the manipulation of an environment aimed at the control—even the eradication—of an insect has taken place.

If the species of tsetse fly seem hard to sort out, those one-celled protozoa, the auger-shaped trypanosomes, are worse. When Bruce and Castellani first saw them they could barely recognize this broad group of organisms from other protozoa. Today one can differentiate many trypanosome species; seven of those which cause disease are associated with tsetse flies. Four of these seven are agents either of nagana or sleeping sickness.

Trypanosomes cause several different diseases of man and animals in the New World and in Asia as well as in Africa; thus today they have a geographical range far greater than tsetse's (see Table 1). Fossil remains of the fly have been found preserved in the shales of Colorado, and some specialists have speculated that in earlier geological times it transmitted trypanosomes to eohippus, an early fox-sized ancestor of the horse, and caused its extinction in the New World.

In South America the species *Trypanasoma cruzi* causes Chagas' disease, which damages the heart muscle of human beings. This trypanosome poses a threat to 35 million people in Latin America. The "kissing bug," *Rhodnius prolixus,* not tsetse, transmits it. *R. prolixus* resembles a cockroach with long and slender legs. During its lifespan of six to ten months, its diet consists mostly of the vital fluids of other insects, but it also feeds upon the American opossum and other mammals, which, like human beings, may harbor the parasite, *T. cruzi.*

R. prolixus, a true bug, "fills itself with human blood which has the effect of making it defecate and so the parasite is deposited on the human skin. If the person then scratches himself the parasite enters the body."

Within two weeks of the parasite's entry, fever begins, and inflammation of the heart muscle and enlargement of the heart ensue. These symptoms may go unnoticed for years. The chronic heart disturbances, however, may lead to premature death. Charles Darwin was bitten by this insect and perhaps infected by this parasite in his visits to Brazil and Argentina on the voyage of the *Beagle.* The lethargy and malaise he experienced in his later life, contrasting with his earlier strength and vigor, have sometimes been attributed to hypochondria, but they may well have been caused by Chagas' disease.

Table 1. Principal species of trypanosomes affecting man and beasts: Their mode of transmission and their geographical distribution

Trypanosome	Disease	Range	Mammalian hosts
Maturation in tsetse flies			
(Stomach and salivary glands)			
T. gambiense	Chronic sleeping sickness	Central Africa	Man
T. rhodesiense	Acute sleeping sickness	East Africa	Man, bovines, antelopes
T. brucei	Nagana	Tropical Africa	All domestic mammals, antelopes
(Proboscis and stomach)			
T. congolense	Nagana	Tropical Africa	Ruminants,* pigs, dogs, equines
T. simiae	Acute or chronic disease	Tropical Africa	Monkeys, pigs, warthogs; possibly bovines, equines, camels
(Proboscis)			
T. vivax	Souma	Central and South America	Ruminants,* equines, dogs
T. uniforme	Relapsing fever, occasionally fatal	East and Central Africa; Angola	Ruminants *
Maturation in kissing bugs (triatomids)			
(Stomach)			
T. cruzi	Chagas disease	Americas: 30° south– 19° north	Armadillo, man
Mechanical transmission by blood-sucking flies other than tsetse			
T. equiperdum	Dourine	South America; North, South and SW Africa	Equines
T. evansi	Surra	North and NW Africa, Sudan, Somalia—all continents	Ruminants,* equines, dogs, monkeys, elephants, etc.

* Cattle, sheep, goats, antelopes, camels.

Performance, more than appearance, distinguishes one species of trypanosome from another. *T. brucei* and *T. congolense* will infect dogs, but *T. brucei* also will infect horses and *T. congolense* will produce disease in ruminants and pigs; *T. gambiense* and *T. rhodesiense* infect man. Some people speculate that *T. rhodesiense* is really an ancestral trypanosome derived from *T. brucei* and that *T. rhodesiense* gave rise to *T. gambiense*. Others believe that it is instead a particularly virulent offshoot of *T. gambiense*. Whatever their relationship actually happens to be, until recently only their comparative virulence in causing sleeping sickness and *T. rhodesiense*'s resistance to arsenical drugs used in treating patients separated the one from the other.

Most trypanosomes are cyclical, which is to say that in their insect host they undergo transformation. This transformation or change in shape can happen in the insect proboscis, in the stomach and the proboscis, or, as in the case of trypanosomes that cause sleeping sickness and nagana, in the stomach and the salivary glands of tsetse. The trypanosomes reach the stomach of tsetse in long and slender form, but as they pass upward through the insect tissue to the salivary glands they fatten, shorten, and become infective forms. Bruce and Castellani did not realize that trypanosomes could be cyclical when they first saw them. They thought that transmission of the disease was by direct means. And it is true that mechanical transmission can take place, though it rarely does, through the bite of a fly that has recently drawn blood from an infected animal or person. Alternatively, a man can be bitten by a fly and not contract sleeping sickness because the trypanosomes that the fly may be harboring have not matured and reached the salivary glands. Dr. F. K. Kleine, a German working in Tanganyika in 1908, observed the changes these parasites undergo during the three weeks they spend in tsetse before these flies let them go to man and beast. He realized that the trypanosomes had to pass

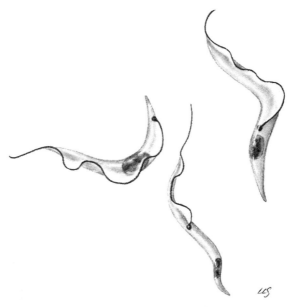

Trypanosomes as they occur in the tsetse fly. (Drawn by Lonna Lagreco Scott.)

through this maturation process in order to become infective.

Kleine, then, on the eve of World War I had closed the last major gap in knowledge of the intricate relationships among hosts, parasites, and vectors. The fly was now known to transmit the trypanosomes which caused nagana in cattle and sleeping sickness in man. Men realized also that these trypanosomes underwent a maturation process within the fly before they could be infective to their hosts, whether man or beast. Later workers would pull together many of the loose ends of these fundamental discoveries. But sufficient information was now at hand so that man could intelligently combat the fly and the trypanosomes.

This opportunity for action fired the imagination of the public and replaced or supplemented the drama of the fundamental discoveries. In the process of this change in emphasis a new profession, medical entomology, gained impetus. Here, as in the fight against malaria, yellow fever, elephantiasis, and other insect-transmitted diseases, the doctor and the entomologist had to work together. They had to marshal all the resources possible to combat the insect and the diseases it transmitted if success was to be achieved.

Campaigns against
Tsetse and Trypanosomes

*None the less, he knew that the tale he had to tell could not be
one of a final victory. It could be only the record of what had
had to be done, and what assuredly would have to be done again
in the never ending fight against terror and its relentless onslaughts,
despite their personal afflictions, by all who, while unable to be
saints but refusing to bow down to pestilences, strive their utmost
to be healers.*

Albert Camus
The Plague

By the early twentieth century, scientists had discovered the
cause of human and animal trypanosomiasis and the agent,
tsetse, which spread it; they were busy filling in the chinks of
their knowledge. They then could and did devise ways to apply
this knowledge and suppress the disease.

A few broad strategies seemed obvious to harassed administrators who possessed a few important facts about flies and parasites and who were confronted with a major epidemic like the
one which gripped East Africa from 1895 to 1905. One such
plan of action was aimed mainly toward potential human victims and was designed to break their contact with the fly. This
required administrative skill; it meant reorganizing people
within the fly belts or removing people from these areas alto-

gether. Another strategy was pointed primarily at the fly, to remove it from the places men and animals needed to occupy. This could be done simply by catching flies by hand or in traps or by altering the habitat they needed in which to survive and to reproduce. Only later would chemical warfare with DDT and its relatives become possible. The third strategy, medical in nature, was directed against the trypanosomes. The disease could be conquered by treating multitudes of infected people and livestock, not only to cure each of them of the disease, but also, by curing them, to destroy the trypanosomes throughout these major sources of the fly's food. A fourth strategy was directed toward eliminating wild animals, the natural reservoir of trypanosomes and a source of food for tsetse.

Many different environments harbored different species of fly across the broad span of Africa, and there were many different patterns of human behavior and different interrelations of fly, trypanosome, and host. Different strategies were therefore emphasized in different combinations in accordance with the times, the places, and the state of knowledge about the fly and the trypanosomes. Doctors, entomologists, and administrators, among others, grasped at each new straw of knowledge. Eager for the panacea of control or eradication of this pest and disease, they often so stressed a particular new strategy or tactic that it assumed a voracious life of its own. They failed to recognize that strategies or tactics of pest and disease control needed to be in harmony with the lives of the people and that they must not destroy the integrity of the land.

The long-range result, however, was a dramatic decline of the diseases almost everywhere. Complications arose, of course, such as the appearance of a virulent new trypanosome which caused the Rhodesian form of sleeping sickness, the spread of flies and parasites to new areas, the development of resistance to drugs among the trypanosomes, the rising costs of labor when the early control methods required man-hours in the thousands, and the difficulty local people experienced in understanding the importance of measures imposed on them from above. As a result the victory was not complete, and the campaign was marked by many setbacks.

Since it was the sleeping sickness epidemic in East Africa that had shocked colonial administrators into action and had led to the discoveries we have just described, it was naturally here that the first strategies were devised. Robert Koch, working in the Sese Islands off the shores of German East Africa, now Tanzania, in Lake Victoria, for example, learned that *Glossina palpalis* favored the blood of crocodiles, and he proposed that these reptiles be killed off. His suggestion was not adopted, however, and in the main the Germans relied on the treatment of sleeping sickness victims till the end of World War I, when they lost the territory to the British.

British-administered Uganda, however, had a new commissioner who saw a more direct way to break the man-fly contact in the lakeshore areas where fly eradication seemed hopeless. This civil servant was Hesketh Bell, who had served in a number of junior posts in the colonial service in the West Indies and as administrator for the island of Dominica in the Windwards. A prolific author, he wrote on his experiences in the West Indies under such titles as *Love in Black* and *A Witch's Legacy.*

His *Glimpses of a Governor's Life,* based on his diary, is rich with anecdotes about that period when the epidemic of sleeping sickness was raging in Uganda. From his writings Bell emerges at times as a man impressed with his own importance and certainly as one with a flair for the dramatic. He thought, for instance, that the African people might remember him, if for no other reason, because he rode an elephant. No African could do this; African elephants are too wild. But Bell imported an Indian elephant for the purpose. His riding an elephant caused more excitement among the local people than the arrival of the telephone and the telegraph. But another, more important aspect of Bell's personality shines through his works. During his three-year administration, first as commissioner, then as governor of the Protectorate of Uganda, he operated as a forceful and determined executive who took personal interest in breaking man-fly contact to eliminate sleeping sickness.

In 1907, Bell proposed that all the people, sick and well, be moved far enough away from the shores of Lake Victoria to be out of reach of the fly. He reasoned that without sufficient man-fly intimacy the trypanosome population would play out as the flies that carried them died. Later the people would be able to reenter the area and live with the fly with impunity.

Time after time Bell asked the Colonial Office (which had taken over responsibility for governing Uganda from the Foreign Office in 1905) for authority to order the chiefs and their people to retreat from the fly-infested regions. The Colonial Office would not give it to him. In London men deemed his plan too expensive, too drastic.

Bell quietly took matters into his own hands; he ordered the chiefs to move their people and the villages to higher land away from the fly haunts. The people complied and the epidemic subsided. When Bell went to London further to plead his case he still received negative reactions. Later, in *Glimpses of a Governor's Life,* Bell wrote:

Old Sir Partick [Manson] . . . seemed to think that my scheme was not at all a practical one from various points of view. He considered that it would be impossible to remove, more or less forcibly, from their farms and ancestral homes on the lake shore, anything like a 100,000 people and felt sure that we would be let in for a serious native war. He considered that a much better plan would be to clear completely of forest the whole of the fly-infested belt bordering on the lake, especially as that process had proved so successful in the neighborhood of Entebbe.

On my pointing out that such a measure would involve the complete clearance of something like 1,000 square miles of land and an immense expenditure, the Committee agreed with me in thinking that this would not be a practical measure. After a good deal of rather desultory talking I decided that the moment had come for telling them what the present situation actually is. I said, "Gentlemen, I am glad to be able to tell you that some of you are arguing against what is a *fait accompli*. Considering the terrible mortality that was constantly increasing and the fact that there appeared, so far, to be no therapeutic remedy, I felt that something drastic must be done at once. I have therefore taken upon myself the responsibility of going ahead with the measures that I recommended in my despatch, and am happy to say that, already, almost half of the fly-infested lake shore has been completely cleared of its inhabitants and that they have been settled in fly-free areas."

I told them that, barring one small affray in one village in which three people were wounded, there has not been the slightest conflict with the people. The Chiefs, realizing that the intentions of the government are for the good of their tenants, have most loyally assisted us, and have already helped to provide some of the camps required for the segregation of the thousands of infected people who, unless a cure be soon found, are bound to die. If the Imperial Treasury will provide the funds required for continuing and completing these measures, I have every reason to hope that the results will be successful, and that, after a certain number of years, the tsetse fly, being unable to renew its supply of infection, will become as harmless as it was before Sleeping Sickness appeared in the country. It should then be possible to restore the people to their homes and farms on the lake shore.

The result of my statement was wonderful. I was heartily congratulated on what we had already done and was assured that the

Committee would recommend that all the funds required for the prosecution of the plan should be provided. I left the C.O. feeling very happy.

Thus one early broad attack on human trypanosomiasis in Africa involved a wholesale movement of human population. This weapon was based on the knowledge that the fly that carried the disease occupied a limited and easily recognized type of habitat.

Bell calculated correctly that moving people away from the fly belt would effectively break the man-trypanosome contact because it would separate man from the fly. He erred, however, in assuming that the people could move back to their shoreline homes and live there with impunity after the trypanosomes had played out of the fly population. He did not know that the Gambian trypanosomes could live and multiply in game. Nevertheless, moving people from fly-infested areas and a method mentioned in the quotation above, the clearing of forest, were applied widely in the battle against the disease in the decade to come. The method foreshadowed by Koch, game eradication, also came into wide play.

In November 1907, Winston Churchill, then a prominent member of Parliament, traveled in East Africa. His mission was a personal one, "for the formation of opinion, for the stirring and enlivenment of thought, and for the discernment of colour and proportion" which he believed were priceless gifts of travel. Churchill arrived in Uganda "in white uniform and a galaxy of medals," as Bell described him, "and was received by a Guard of Honour of the Indian troops."

At first he pictured the Kingdom of Uganda as "a fairy tale. You climb up a railway instead of a beanstalk, and at the end there is a wonderful new world." Later he noted among other "malignant attributes" the insidious toll insects which transmit diseases were taking, and he stated "Uganda is defended by its insects." Reviewing at first hand the tsetse situation, Churchill succinctly articulated the state of war against tsetse and in a wider sense the standard pattern of a campaign against any pest. He wrote in *My African Journey:* "International Commissions discuss him [tsetse] round green tables, grave men peer patiently at him through microscopes, active officers scour Central Africa to plot him out on charts. A fine-spun net is being woven remorselessly around him."

A few years after Hesketh Bell's unauthorized solution to the Uganda epidemic, the government of Portugal was forced to act against sleeping sickness in one of its tiniest possessions, fifty-eight-square-mile Príncipe Island. Located in the Gulf of Guinea just 160 miles from Rio Muni in West Africa, this island had become infested, probably around 1825, with tsetse fly from the continent, and the trypanosome had entered perhaps from the western region of Gabon, from the Congo, or from Portuguese Angola, from which laborers were brought to the island to work on the plantations. The fly found a flourishing and satisfactory life with the help of the wild pigs that abounded in the forest, and the disease spread through the human population until it threatened the island's viability and brought outcries from other countries similar to those that had forced King Leopold II of the Belgians to institute reforms in the Congo. But Príncipe, unlike the vast continent, had a limited area and population which made feasible the goal of complete eradication of both fly and parasite. The methods designed to achieve this end were often employed in Africa in other campaigns.

Two Portuguese explorers, Joã de Santarém and Pedro Escobar, had discovered the island on St. Anthony's day, January 17, 1471, and named it after that saint. In 1500 the island was given to a Portuguese nobleman, António Carneiro, on the con-

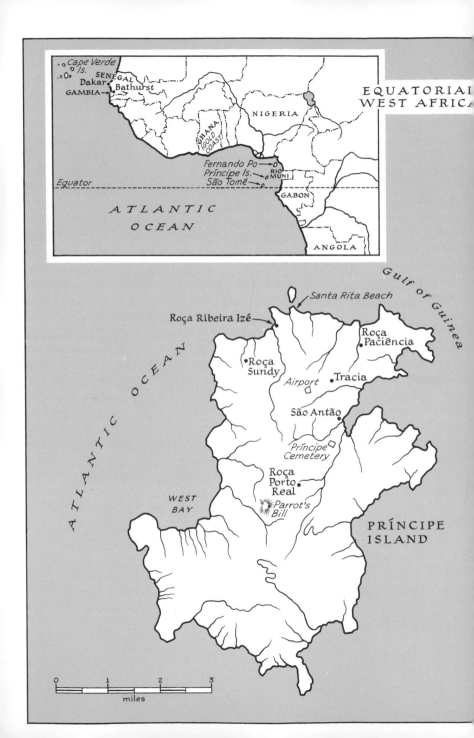

EQUATORIAL
WEST AFRICA

Cape Verde Is.
Dakar
SENEGAL
GAMBIA   Bathurst

NIGERIA

GHANA
(GOLD COAST)

Fernando Po
Príncipe Is.
São Tomé

RIO MUNI

Equator

GABON

ATLANTIC OCEAN

ANGOLA

Gulf of Guinea

Santa Rita Beach
Roça Ribeira Izé
Roça Paciência
Roça Sundy
Airport
Tracia
São Antão
Príncipe Cemetery
Roça Porto Real
Parrot's Bill

ATLANTIC OCEAN

WEST BAY

PRÍNCIPE ISLAND

0   1   2   3
miles

dition that one-tenth of the produce therefrom be reserved for Prince D. João. On that account it became known as Príncipe, or Prince's Island. Sugarcane from Madeira was introduced in 1502, and for the next two hundred years its cultivation was the island's main industry. In 1690 a newly founded organization, the Cacheu and Cabo Verde Company, developed a shipping traffic which flourished and brought prosperity to the island because it was on the cattle and slave trade route from Africa to Brazil. But by 1811 this traffic was declining rapidly, and island commerce went bankrupt. Even as late as 1855, when the island was regaining prosperity from a growing cacao and coffee trade, Dr. Thomas J. Hutchinson, senior surgeon of the steamship *Pleiad,* could report about the island capital, St. Antonio: "All the shops appear as if a ray of blessed sunshine never crossed their doorways, to dazzle the moths and spiders in their dark retreats."

Hutchinson's *Pleiad,* returning from an exploration of the Niger River in West Africa, had anchored at Príncipe because its engine had failed and the crew needed to take on more provisions for the long trip home under sails, which had thoughtfully been provided just for such an eventuality. Geese, turkeys, fowl, goats, and a few pigs with sharp backs and long snouts were brought aboard. Like the rats in Albert Camus' Algerian city of Oran, beset physically and symbolically with bubonic plague, the pigs of Príncipe were the key to the generation of a pestilence—sleeping sickness—on the island. Moreover, the pigs—unlike the rats, which died of the plague—lived on and on to harbor the parasites of sleeping sickness.

At about this time the island's mistress was Dona Maria Correia, a woman whom one may imagine as he pleases because a haze of history so completely enshrouds her. She could have been a petite, vivacious, young Portuguese princess, a royal person who by a series of land grants inherited this tropi-

Príncipe Island. (Drawn by John Morris.)

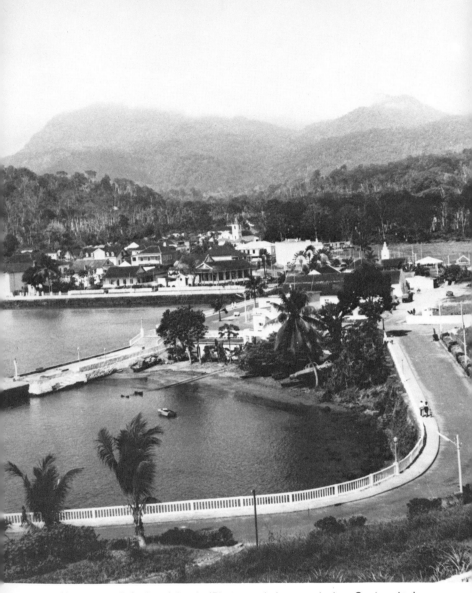

Harbor on Príncipe Island. (Photograph by permission Centro de Informaçao e Turismo, S. Tomé e Príncipe.)

cal isle that impressed sailors as a "colossal bouquet of greenery emerging direct from the ocean." If she had been like
many other heirs of vast estates in Portuguese realms, she
would have lived behind a façade of *azulejos* (blue tiles) in a
Lisbon palace, perhaps regretting that her bequest had not been
a nearby estate of wheat, vineyards, and olive trees, and she
would have visited her island infrequently. A shadowy figure
about whom little is known despite the fact that she owned
practically all the land, Dona Maria lived on the island in pala-
tial homes and prospered from obscure varieties of trade as
well as by the cultivation of her lands.

In 1841, fourteen years prior to the visit of the *Pleiad,* Captain William Allen and Dr. T. R. H. Thomson, also on a return
trip from an expedition to the Niger River which Captain H.
D. Trotter commanded, put in at Príncipe's West Bay to refuel.

[They] were much struck with the beauty and singularity of the
bold peaks, clothed with wood to the very summit. Among these
the "Parrot's Bill" is the most remarkable, shooting up like a gigantic crystal from the dense forest. . . .

The climate is unhealthy even for the natives, except in December, January, and February, when it is comparatively dry; though
at West Bay it is said there is no day throughout the year without
rain. Heavy mists sweeping round the lofty peaks give additional
grandeur, and make them sometimes appear as if overhanging the
bay. After curling and playing about the ravines of the mountains,
these mists suddenly descend, and deluge the shores.

Príncipe they said, "may truly be called the 'watery gem of the
ocean.' "

Allen and Thomson met a Madame Ferreira. Could she
have been Dona Maria Correia? The names are easy to confuse. Moreover, a Don Fernando Correia Henriques de No-
ronha had served as provisional governor in 1836. They go on
in their tale of their visit to Príncipe Island:

We arranged with Madame Ferreira for a supply of firewood, which she keeps ready cut for the cruisers on the coast, at the rate of one hundred billets for a dollar.

This lady, of Portuguese parents, was the widow of the late governor, who was previously judge. With the laudable intention of introducing improvements in the cultivation and management of her estates, on her return to Prince's from a visit to Europe, she brought with her a numerous suite of white persons and their families, among whom fever soon however, made fearful ravages. Two remarkably handsome Spanish boys, like the finest conceptions of Murillo, had, since their arrival, lost their father, mother, a brother and a sister. The European gardener, his wife and three daughters, as well as the young daughter of M. Fretus, Madame Ferreira's factotum, were lying ill with the fever. The latter we saw lying on a couch—a most interesting and picturesque object.

This enterprising lady seemed most anxious to carry into effect numerous plans for the benefit of the island, and had commenced by erecting mills for sugar, oil, and for sawing timber. Abundance of seeds brought from Spain flourished among the rocks in the garden around her house, mingled with beautiful indigenous flowers. All her property in West Bay she was desirous of selling to the English Government, alleging the persecutions of the Governor of the island, who had involved her in many lawsuits on charges— whether just or unjust we could not ascertain—of being engaged in the slave trade. However this may be, the English officers belonging to the squadron have ever been received by her with great hospitality and kindness.

If Dona Maria Correia, like Madame Ferreira, had been a widow of a crown servant, she would have been entitled to a dowry constituting leases on crown land valid for three generations provided she lived on the island to see to it that the land was cultivated and that the right of inheritance descended to her children and grandchildren. She would then have been considered part of the fixed population of the island, a native, or *filha da terra*—a category whose population approximated 3,000 in the nineteenth century and was distinguished from a larger population of transients and immigrants regarded as "floaters." By 1907 the "natives" had dwindled to 350, decimated as they were by sleeping sickness, malaria, and other tropical diseases.

About seventy years after Allen and Thompson met Madame Ferreira, Dr. Bernardo Francisco Bruto da Costa, a member of one of the Portuguese commissions investigating sleeping sickness, met Manoel dos Santos Abreu, the administrator in charge of the Porto Real estates in central Príncipe. He told Bruto da Costa that Dona Maria Correia had possessed magnificent palaces in the northern and eastern part of the island. A church which she built but which had gone to ruin on the estate Ribeira Izé attested to her affluence. She used that estate, he said, as her favorite home and as a checking station for the slaves and cattle from Angola and Gabon, in which "merchandise" she did a thriving business as these were sent to Brazil. Flat-bottomed boats handled the traffic in cattle and slaves. They were easy to beach in the shallow bay at the estate. Abreu probably got most of his information from Delfina, Dona Maria's goddaughter (daughter of Madame Ferreira's factotum?), who died on the island about 1912.

Filipe Xavier Paixão, an aged native crewman of one of the flat-bottomed boats, also told Abreu that tsetse was not known on the island before it served as a "rest stop" for those slaves who were to be transported to the New World. He said that tsetse came with the slaves and the cattle from Angola, the Gold Coast, and especially Gabon on the western coast of Africa. The Portuguese called the fly Mosca do Gabão, their name for the species *Glossina palpalis*. Bruto da Costa reported that according to local tradition it had arrived on the island about 1825. It would seem, then, that a large part of the responsibility for the introduction and establishment of the tsetse might really have devolved on Dona Maria or Madame Ferreira. It could have reached the island even earlier, of course. The Cacheu and Cabo Verde Company, which also trafficked in cattle and slaves, would then have had to share the blame. In any case, once the Mosca do Gabão arrived, the island possessed the basic material for sleeping sickness infections, pigs as host and flies as vector just as Camus' Oran possessed rats and fleas as instruments for the transmission to man of the bacillus that causes bubonic plague.

Suddenly, probably during Dona Maria's lifetime, the trypanosome causing sleeping sickness arrived and the disease broke out. The first person known to have died from it was a slave buried there in July 1859. As written in the record of burials:

Yesterday at seven o'clock p.m. died Mariana Manoel, slave woman belonging to Manoel Rodrigues Pedronho, from the sickness "Sinolência" (Sleepiness), according to the Physician. Born in Costa. Age 50. Will be buried in due place without a coffin at ten o'clock a.m. Paid the sum of 700 "reis." Principe Island cemetery on July 9th, 1859. Cintra, President. Receipt for 200 "reis." Teves Regedor Damiao Vaz Pauleth.

Several other deaths from sleeping sickness were reported that year.

Toward the close of the nineteenth century cacao had replaced coffee as the principal crop, but the estates still required ever-increasing numbers of laborers. They were conscripted from Angola, Cape Verde, and Gabon on contracts extending for two, three, or (before 1903) five years. These laborers— over three thousand strong—constituted the largest element of the early-twentieth-century floating population. They, too, probably brought sleeping-sickness trypansomes with them; the *palpalis* species of tsetse fed readily on these men. The fly may have missed its favorite species of wildlife, particularly the crocodile, but it adjusted quite well to the limited diet of domestic and wild pigs, dogs, cattle, civet cats, and human beings, and, to a much lesser extent if at all, to monkeys, rats, and bats, which also occupied the island.

Lowest in status, highest in economic worth because they worked, the non-European floaters, the laborers, held the key to the welfare of the island. As sleeping sickness picked these people off, the great cacao estates became uneconomic to manage for want of labor. Moral issues as well as economic ones flared up. The disease, together with the poor working conditions, caused such a high mortality that English merchants who bought much of the cacao became alarmed. W. A. Cadbury, among other prosperous English Quakers, refused to purchase cacao coming from this island or from São Tomé or Angola until the Portuguese government took steps to improve the working conditions of the laborers, which meant doing some thing about sleeping sickness. He, his company, and others turned to the Gold Coast, now Ghana, where production of cacao beans for the chocolate industry was vested in the hands of many local people rather than a few estate owners. Whether or not the boycott had any effect, the Portuguese, faced with a prosperous agriculture on the verge of ruin, were forced in 1911 to set about ridding the island of sleeping sickness and the fly.

To eradicate tsetse and the disease took the efforts of three sleeping sickness commissions extending over fifteen years. The costs of the major campaign from 1911 to 1914 ran to approximately $275,000, borne by the planters and the state.

The first Portuguese sleeping sickness commission (1901) ante-dated the drive to eradicate tsetse from Príncipe. It preceded the commissions that the English formed in Uganda and was constituted even before Dr. Jack Cook's article appeared formally to announce the presence of sleeping sickness in that land. The members of this commission stopped only briefly on the island in May 1901; their primary interest was to assess the seriousness of the disease in Angola. But on Príncipe the commission described six clinical cases which probably came from the hospital on Roça Sundy estate close to Ribeira Izé, Dona Maria's favorite estate, and spotted the bacterium in spinal fluid that brought them into a dispute with Castellani. They also collected data on the mortality from the disease, but the state of knowledge was too rudimentary at that time for the commission to recommend practical control measure. Dr. Corrêa Mendes took part in the mission; Professor Annibal Bettencourt headed it.

Corrêa Mendes led the second commission, which worked on the island in 1907 and 1908. This group made a complete study of the local epidemic, depicted the poor sanitary conditions there, and planned a strategy for fly and disease control which marshaled all available facts about tsetse and its trypanosomes discovered in other parts of Africa as well as in Príncipe. The strategy recommended included five methods of attack—taping gluey black cloths to the clothes worn by working men to attract and to kill the flies and thus reduce their numbers, using arsenic to clear trypanosomes from the blood of infected people, clearing land to keep flies away from habitations, corralling domesticated stock, and—most effective of all —killing wild pigs, the flies' favorite host, and all other wild game upon which the fly fed.

The second commission returned to Portugal in September 1908 and shortly afterward presented its recommendations to the government. Not until early in 1911, more than two years later, did the government attempt to enforce them, but in the meantime on a hit-or-miss basis the methods of attack they had recommended came into practice as control measures of desperation.

The third sleeping sickness commission grew from the need to put teeth into the recommendations of the second. It became obvious that all planters on the island were not going to implement these recommendations voluntarily and that the implementation would not be enough even if they did. Thus on April 17, 1911, the Portuguese government by decree gave force of law to the Corrêa Mendes mission's recommendations and instituted a sleeping sickness commission made up of the administrator of the council, the health officer, the president of the municipality, and two planters.

The method of trapping flies on sticky clothes originated from a device that Bulhões Maldonado, administrator of Roça Sundy, had used in 1906. Maldonado had outfitted several of his workers with dark-colored cloths forty by fifty centimeters in size smeared with a gooey paste of palm oil and pine resin. They wore these cloths on their backs as they were at work cutting grass. Over a twenty-month period they attracted to them 133,778 flies, which liked the dark color. This method seemed so promising that it received official sanction as a campaign measure in 1911. At first, all laborers on all the estates were supposed to wear a white outfit with a contrasting black "sticky cloth" and in addition a light hood over the head with a flap to cover the nape of the neck to ward off the flies. Later the official number of those who were required to wear this garb was reduced to 10 percent.

The last commission had authority to deploy sanitary brigades into the bush. It hoped that the men of these brigades wearing sticky cloths would attract such tremendous numbers of flies that the insect's population would drop below the level it required to sustain itself. The first brigade consisted of forty-three persons, all prisoners of war from São Tomé and delinquents sentenced to penal servitude. The cloths were of black serge because the flies preferred to alight on black objects, and the gooey substance in this case was a "rat varnish" imported from England; it was the color of honey and a little thicker, was very sticky, and smelled not of resin but of linseed oil.

The system worked up to a point but no further. While two men wearing sticky cloths could collect from 1,500 to 2,000 insects in the first few days of a campaign in one area, the number would diminish to twenty at the end of a week's work, and an irreducible population of flies would get by and survive.

The Maldonado method had other disadvantages—it was cumbersome, the wearer tired readily, and the gluey matter had to be reapplied daily. Although flies were scraped off and counted each day, the addition of fresh layers built up on the cloth until the clothing itself weighed six to eight pounds. When the wearers penetrated lands as yet uncleared, leaves and debris stuck to their clothing and nullified its effectiveness. The Portuguese themselves really did not consider that the use of sticky cloths afforded the final solution for exterminating flies. Bruto da Costa pointed out that sticky cloths did, however, protect workers in areas of high fly density and did give a reasonably good index of fly population.

While the brigades were trapping flies, Portuguese doctors, following the work of Bruce, the Cook brothers, Koch, and Ayres Kopke in Lisbon, were relying on arsenic in the form of atoxyl to kill the trypanosomes. The members of the second Portuguese commission had already worked out a double-injection technique—two inoculations of 0.5 or 0.6 gram of atoxyl at forty-eight-hour intervals every two weeks for a period of six months. Later, persons bitten by the fly were required to report to the doctors for a preventive dose of atoxyl within twenty-four hours after having been bitten. Finally the time lapse between bite and injection was telescoped to seven hours. Doctors administered nearly 100 pounds of atoxyl in these ways from 1907 to the end of the campaign—enough for 75,000 partial doses of 0.6 gram. Three times between 1911 and 1914 virtually the whole population of the island, nearly four thousand inhabitants, passed for review for the examination of their blood and for treatment where necessary. The entire domestic animal population had to submit to the same regimen of examination and to treatment if infection was discovered.

The incidence of sleeping sickness dropped, but the attack against the trypanosomes did not stamp out the disease. Campaigners had to intensify their efforts to wipe out the fly; hence another prong of attack, and perhaps the most important one —to starve out the fly population by separating it from its hosts was initiated. The margins of land around houses had to be cleared to keep the fly back from habitations. It was compulsory to clear secondary jungle growth and forests where the fly abounded and where contact with people and domestic animals would occur. All dwellings of staff and establishments for Europeans or natives had to have screens on windows and doors. When working in the fields, laborers had to wear light-colored clothing covering the body to the wrists and ankles, and cloth of similar color over the head. Draft animals, when not at work, were also protected by screened enclosures, and no dog who had a master who cared about him could roam during the daytime when the fly was active.

Finally, the authorities enforced a decree issued in February 1911, before the formation of the third commission; this decree forbade the rearing of pigs, to which the flies had become especially attracted. The decree instructed those who had stocks of pigs to destroy them. Some plantation owners and managers complied; others decided they could beat the game by releasing their swine to run wild. They could then depend upon these hogs as a source of meat without legal penalty for keeping them penned. This action hampered the work of the brigades that were deployed throughout the island to clear the jungle and to exterminate all pigs, dogs, and civet cats, but the extermination campaign went on. As the number of pigs on the island diminished, the numbers of flies per pig increased remarkably. Like the flies, the pigs had a residual population that became increasingly difficult to ferret out and remove as a major source of food for the fly.

Stray dogs also presented a problem; by the time the campaign was over, two thousand had been executed. About the same number of civet cats were killed. Tsetse could not even go to monkeys—a casual host—because monkeys had been virtually exterminated for quite a different reason: they damaged the crops.

Divested of its sources of food, the tsetse population finally played out. In early 1914 only thirty-four flies could be found on the whole island; the last one was caught in April. Later that year it became impossible to find a single fly, and for forty-two years Dona Maria's island maintained its freedom from the scourge of tsetse and its trypanosomes and regained a measure of prosperity as a source of cacao.

Members of the three sleeping sickness commissions who did their work so well on Príncipe must have left the island with a great sense of satisfaction for a job well done. Perhaps as practicing scientists and medical men they also experienced a certain humbleness about their accomplishments, as did Dr. Rieux in Camus' story of the plague. Perhaps they knew that sleeping sickness might bide its time and return to the island at some later date and that their story could also be only "the record of what had had to be done, and what assuredly would have to be done again in the never ending fight against terror and its relentless onslaughts."

Inevitably, in the 1950's tsetse reinvaded Príncipe. If one could read purpose into the actions of a fly, he might almost say it did so with an "I shall return" vindictiveness. These flies came to the attention of Decio Passos, the meteorological observer at the airport on the island, who forwarded one batch to

Portugal. The owner of Roça Sundy also discovered tsetse on Príncipe, and he personally carried another small batch of flies to the director of the Zoological Centre of the Overseas Research Council in Lisbon. From these specimens a veterinarian, Dr. João Tendeiro, identified *Glossina palpalis*. On order from the Overseas Minister, the Council and the Institute of Tropical Medicine in Lisbon immediately dispatched a study team headed by Professor João Fraga de Azevedo to spend three months investigating the new outbreak. They started their work on May 15, 1956, just twelve days after *G. palpalis* was identified.

First, the team asked, did tsetse really reestablish a beach-head on Príncipe or had its evacuation in 1914 been incomplete? Had some tsetse flies survived on the twenty wild swine estimated to have survived the eradication efforts then, when more than 4,500 of these animals were exterminated? Professor Azevedo and his colleagues thought forty years was too long a period of time for the island to have harbored tsetse unnoticed.

It tsetse arrived anew in the 1950's, when and from where could it have come? All direct communications between Príncipe and tsetse-infested areas elsewhere had ceased except for those between that island and Fernando Po, known to harbor tsetse flies. About thirty boats per year stopped at Príncipe, but they came from Cape Verde and went to São Tomé or vice versa. Planes brought passengers and cargo from Fernando Po to Príncipe monthly, and the trip took no more than one and a half hours. Fernando Po was obviously the most likely source of the new tsetse infestation.

To establish when tsetse arrived proved to be a difficult task indeed. Azevedo's team interviewed 3,095 people—very nearly all the adults on the island. Two hundred and ninety of them said tsetse was there in 1956; no one had noticed it before September 1955.

Tidbits of information, however, began to appear. The administrator in Roça Paciência said that at the close of 1954 "many of his men were pestered by 'a much stinging fly.' " A Mr. Cupertino who lived in the village of Tracia, where the flies were especially numerous in May of 1956, said that one day when "his wife was pregnant she went down to the brook which flowed near his home . . . to do her laundry. Once she was stung by a 'strange fly' which gorged itself and caused her a very marked local irritation with oedema and painful itching," the typical symptoms of a tsetse fly bite. From her son's age Professor Azevedo could readily estimate that tsetse had bitten her sometime about 1954. And an old fisherman who had experienced the epidemic at the beginning of the century said that tsetse had appeared again on Santa Rita beach soon after the president of Portugal, Craveiro Lopes, paid a visit in May 1954.

As professors are wont to do, Azevedo theorized about the population buildup of the fly and about whether the population density, as they found it, meant that fly number one really did reach the island in 1954. Starting with a female fly capable of laying six to ten larvae in its lifetime, which is sixty to seventy days under the best conditions, a progression would result in "328 tsetses after one year, 86,127 after 2 years, 14,294,353 after 3 years, . . . 1,595,249,851 after 4 years." In the two-month period from May 17 to July 17, 1956, Azevedo and his companions captured 66,894 flies. From their catches they extrapolated that within a year about 22 million flies and after two years more than 5.5 billion flies would inhabit the island. Somehow these figures indicated to them that 1954 was a very likely year for the reinvasion of Príncipe to have taken place.

Much more important, Azevedo's fly catches and calculations clearly indicated that the increase in the fly population was indeed explosive. In May 1955 a European party had picnicked "quite comfortably on Ribeira Izé Beach, while in April 1956" stinging swarms of flies, later realized to be tsetse, drove a similar party away. In the three months that the Azevedo commission spent on the island, they outlined and started to implement a campaign to eradicate tsetse. They left behind them a work schedule for a *Glossina* combat team.

The task that the Azevedo commission and the subsequent combat team faced was somewhat easier than that of the earlier sleeping sickness commissions. Azevedo and his colleagues knew which eradication methods would work and which would not from the earlier experience. Moreover, the 1956 campaign had to deal with the flies only, not disease as well. The trypanosomes causing sleeping sickness had not recurred on the island. Azevedo's commission found this out by sampling the blood of practically the entire human population except for infants less than a year old and by taking blood samples of all domestic animals. They also examined 6,500 tsetse flies. No trypanosomes appeared in these samples.

In 1956, Azevedo and his group could adopt control methods that had been developed after the time of the early commissions. One of those was the use of fly traps. Two types, the Harris trap employed so effectively to collect *G. pallidipes* in Zululand and the useful Morris trap that worked well in attracting *G. palpalis* in West Africa—which we shall describe more fully later—helped reduce the tsetse fly population in the heavily infested areas of Príncipe in 1956; as one would expect, the Morris trap collected more tsetse on the island than did the Harris trap because the island was infested with *G. palpalis*. Azevedo immediately ordered hundreds of such traps to be constructed, and before the end of his campaign more than 1,-500 were located in heavily infested parts of the island. These traps enabled fly surveyors to verify where the tsetse concentrations were heaviest. For example, in bush and jungle they found it especially numerous at the laundry pools.

Azevedo also had at his disposal persistent insecticides, DDT for example, to spray along the stream banks and in the swampy areas where *G. palpalis* bred as well as on the domestic animals and on the traps themselves. But here he had to be careful not to overspray or spray in the wrong places, for then his campaign would have run into direct conflict with a biological control program using insect predators against the scale insects of cacao on the island.

The management of the pig problem was also easier. Full knowledge of the habits of *G. palpalis* in 1956 enabled Azevedo quite successfully to make a recommendation opposite to Bruto da Costa's in 1912–1914. He could tell the estate owners to corral their pigs and keep them free of flies. Those not corralled, of course, had to be killed. The estate owners no longer had reason to release their swine to roam the bush, and the wild pig extermination program which Azevedo's commission undertook was a manageable one.

Did the Portuguese really banish tsetse from Príncipe for the second time? Probably. Will tsetse return? Of course. And the disease too? Naturally. Tsetse and trypanosomes still occupy Gabon, the Congo, and Angola just as they always have, just as they did before they first invaded Príncipe. What were people doing about them during the same period on the mainland of Africa, along the banks of the Ogooué River of Gabon and amid the swamps of the Oubangui and the Chari Rivers, which drain Chad and French Equatorial Africa?

Take away tsetse's deadly weapon, the trypanosome, and nothing remains but a harmless fly with fuzzy feelers and the irritating sort of bite that Livingstone experienced. In depriving tsetse of its trypanosomes by the then-normal technique of poisoning the trypanosomes in the great pool of human blood from which tsetse fed, two men, one a philosopher, the other a man of action, led in saving thousands of lives throughout the entire humid-tropical regions of French-speaking Africa.

The philosopher was Albert Schweitzer, born in 1875 in northern Alsace. He had also prepared himself in theology and in music. In so doing he attempted to quench a thirst for knowledge that was literally to plague him all his life. "In languages and mathematics," Schweitzer wrote of his early life, "it cost me an effort to accomplish anything. But after a time I felt a certain fascination in mastering subjects for which I had no special talent." Still restless after having mastered theology, music, organ building, and philosophy, Schweitzer in his thirtieth year decided to become a jungle doctor. To do so, he had to embark on a seven-year program of studies to qualify in medicine. He believed that he had become too unorthodox in theology to be acceptable as a missionary in the religious sense. This influenced him to turn toward medicine, but he really wanted a job based on actions rather than on words. By 1912 he was in France specializing in tropical medicine, purchasing supplies, and arranging a myriad of other details for his projected career in Africa. The logistics of preparing his trip to Africa annoyed him at first, but later he enjoyed it.

Schweitzer then "made a definite offer to the Paris Missionary Society to come at my own expense to serve its mission field on the River Ogooué from the centrally situated station at Lambaréné." An American missionary and medical man, Dr. Nassau, had established the Lambaréné station in 1876, two years after missionary work began in the Ogooué district and before Gabon had become a French possession. But in 1892 the Paris Missionary Society replaced the Americans, since they could not comply with the French government regulation that all instruction should be given in French.

Although Schweitzer went to Lambaréné in 1913 to build a hospital and to do something about sleeping sickness, before he

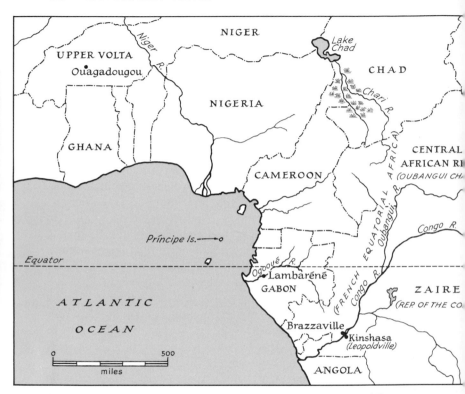

Map of central and western Africa, where Albert Schweitzer and Eugene Jamot worked. (Drawn by John Morris.)

could unpack his drugs and instruments, people suffering from malaria, leprosy, dysentery, pneumonia, and heart disease besieged him, and he had to operate forthwith on patients with strangulated hernias and tumors caused by elephantiasis.

The man of action, Eugène Jamot, also dropped one profession, geology, to take up another, medicine. His first contact with Africa was as an army doctor in Chad in 1911. In 1916, with the power of the French colonial service behind him, he went to Brazzaville on the Congo as director of the Institut Pasteur de Brazzaville to help stamp out sleeping sickness from Equatorial Africa.

Neither Schweitzer nor Jamot did much about the fly itself. To modify the environment, to clear this area of its jungle in order to make it inhospitable to the fly, must have staggered their imaginations if they thought of it at all. They worked exclusively on killing the trypanosomes, first with atoxyl, later with a newer drug called tryparsamide.

The two men used entirely different techniques in their attack on sleeping sickness. Schweitzer zeroed in on one geographical target and physically covered very little of the African continent. Except for an occasional canoe or steamship trip up the Ogooué River or for a fund-raising trip back to Europe, Schweitzer stayed put at Lambaréné, where he ran the village as well as the hospital. He concentrated on the treatment of individual patients, yet the masses flocked to his hospital.

Jamot came to know virtually every bush village of France's equatorial possessions and many of those in West Africa. He cared less, it seemed, about the individual than the masses, yet he ran a campaign in which he and his colleagues ferreted out every individual they could find, afflicted or not with sleeping sickness, from the swamps of the Oubangui-Chari river territory through the arterial waterways of Cameroon to the plains of Ouagadougou in Upper Volta.

Like those before them, Schweitzer and Jamot relied at first on the "frightfully dangerous" atoxyl for treatment of sleeping sickness. It was in the early 1920's that Schweitzer and Jamot tried out the new drug tryparsamide, which was related to atoxyl, on their patients. Under village hospital conditions in a tropical forest setting where logging was the chief industry, Schweitzer administered this arsenical to a timber worker,

N'Tsama, who had an advanced case of sleeping sickness. Like other patients at the stage when the trypanosomes had passed from the bloodstream to the cerebrospinal fluid, N'Tsama, reduced to a skeleton, had an abnormally large appetite and a craving for meat, was highly excitable, showed mental disturbance, and manifested a tendency toward kleptomania. While under treatment with tryparsamide he unfortunately suffered an attack of dysentery and for two months hovered between life and death, so weak that others had to feed him. Schweitzer discontinued the tryparsamide treatments until the approach of spring, when his patient's dysentery subsided. After the treatment was resumed N'Tsama's kleptomania slowly disappeared. He became strong enough to walk, to stand all day by the river bank and fish, and subsequently to lift a heavy plank and carry it away on his head. By summertime N'Tsama asked to be allowed to help with the forest clearing, and except for a certain fatigue this worker was restored to health. He was among the first to show that patients in the last stages of the disease were curable. But N'Tsama never left the hospital community. "The Doctor is my father," he said, "and the hospital is my village."

A German drug called Bayer 205 synthesized in 1916, came into use in the 1920's for treatment of the early stages of sleeping sickness. Schweitzer and others found that tryparsamide was still the most effective drug for advanced cases but that it, like atoxyl, too often damaged the optic nerve and caused partial or complete blindness. In spite of all his care, Schweitzer had one case of blindness from the use of arsenicals to record in his writings in 1930.

Jamot started his campaign in Oubangui-Chari in 1917, when he recruited two European medical men and seven Congolese auxiliaries. The latter could hardly read or write. Jamot and his team possessed three microscopes, two of them probably borrowed, in bad condition, and the third, their own;

six syringes; and two hand centrifuges. By November 1918 the team had five microscopes. Atoxyl was the only medicine effective against sleeping sickness available to the campaigners up to May 1918.

Jamot's plan of action was first to look for suspected cases. All inhabitants of the villages surveyed had to line up for the physician. Each was given a card to be hung around his neck to carry the record of his condition. The suspected cases had to submit to a blood test and if possible (but this was the exception in the bush) to an examination of the spinal fluid. Jamot split his teams into two groups, one to examine, the other to treat, and these teams functioned simultaneously. Using three microscopes, the diagnostic team could examine the blood of eighty to one hundred suspected cases a day. The sick ones received repeated injections of atoxyl at intervals of two to three months.

In the period from August 1917 to May 1919, almost all the villages in Oubangui-Chari from the Oubangui River to the frontier of Chad received visits from Jamot and his coworkers. The people in this area constituted a quarter of the population of Oubangui-Chari, about 100,000 people in an area of about 100,000 square kilometers. Out of 89,643 people examined, 5,347 had sleeping sickness. From these early findings Jamot recommended the assignment of one physician, three European nurses, and ten African nurses for each 50,000 inhabitants to be examined and the creation in each territory of a permanent mission of prophylaxis.

In 1924 and 1925, Jamot systematically examined practically all of the inhabitants in northern Cameroon. He canvased 214 villages housing 14,877 people of whom 1,836 were diseased. As he moved north, he entered the fly territory of *Glossina tachinoides,* the nervous, quick-moving, jittery fly which occupied the same riverine environment as did *G. palpalis.*

The French government established the Permanent Mission of Sleeping Sickness Prophylaxis and appointed Major Jamot as its director in 1926. By that time, Jamot had seven teams directed by physicians prospecting for the disease; each team had eight to fourteen microscopes. A complete map of the disease for the Cameroon was completed in 1928 and the contaminated zones were circumscribed; this area comprised 80,000 square kilometers with a population of 800,000 people.

Physicians, scientists, statisticians, politicians, and others attacked Jamot and his group for their autocratic methods—for trying to establish a state within a state by insisting upon autonomy for the management of the campaign. They argued about the validity of the statistics the teams put forth listing people examined, diseased, and cured. Making allowances for lapses in the best management of these campaigns, one still sees an impressive record of virtual eradication of sleeping sickness from French Equatorial Africa through the method that Jamot devised.

One of the most controversial events in Jamot's life involved the use of tryparsamide. In 1923 he received 250 grams of this new trypanocide from Dr. Louise Pearce of the Rockefeller Institute and Dr. L. M. J. J. Van Hoof, a prominent Belgian worker with whom Dr. Pearce was collaborating. From this amount of chemical, Jamot treated fourteen patients, each of whom received just one injection. As in the case of atoxyl, Jamot, of course, anticipated that an overdose of tryparsamide might damage the eyes of these patients. This did not happen, so he used this chemical more freely in his campaign. Six or seven years later one of Jamot's young, somewhat overzealous and irresponsible aides was working as a doctor in an area of Cameroon where people were seriously afflicted with sleeping sickness. Jamot had been extremely careful in the use of tryparsamide, considering the chemical still in the experimental stage.

His circulars and instructions were clear and precise on the question of dosage—four to six centigrams per kilogram of body weight, for an adult of average weight, with a maximum of three grams per injection. But on his own initiative, this particular doctor instructed his sanitary assistants to administer dosages two to three times the prescribed dose, on the chance that they would be more effective. He began with a dose of 2.5 grams for an adult weighing 60 kilograms, increased it a half a gram for each subsequent injection, and soon was administering doses of from seven to eight grams per injection, which corresponded to ten to fourteen centigrams of tryparsamide per kilogram of body weight, treble the recommended dose. He used this excessive prescription for more than a year. Seven hundred of his patients went blind. The governor of Cameroon removed him from the country. Jamot, feeling sorry for the young doctor, defended him and himself fell under a barrage of criticism that damaged his career and impaired the progress of the campaign. In fact, French authorities arrested Jamot and detained him at Dakar in Senegal for six months, where he could do nothing.

Schweitzer and Jamot each in his own way bequeathed gifts to posterity which they received from the truly tropical tsetse and trypanosome country of Africa. The Ogooué River with all of its physical inconveniences—hot, humid climate, disease, trypanosomes, tsetse flies—afforded Schweitzer a setting for reflection. In September 1915 he was on the deck of a boat steaming up the Ogooué River, thinking and writing, when "late on the third day, at the very moment when, at sunset, we were making our way through a herd of hippopotamuses, there flahsed upon my mind, unforeseen and unsought, the phrase, 'Reverence for Life.' "

The animal husbandman who cares for cattle faces a dilemma similar to Schweitzer's and applies his philosophy "Reverence for Life." He loves his animals, yet he must kill them if he is to live by his occupation. But he does not kill them unnecessarily. Schweitzer says, "I rejoice over the new remedies for sleeping sickness, which enable me to preserve life, whereas I had previously to watch a painful disease. But every time I have under the microscope the germs which cause the disease, I cannot but reflect that I have to sacrifice this life in order to save other life."

Jamot contributed the total approach to a problem, the recognition of its breadth and the invention of strategies to attack it. The forests and swamps of the Oubangui and Chari rivers ordained the population density of that area; they confined the inhabitants in concentrated spots along the water's edge. The swamps likewise enabled tsetse to capitalize on its ability to transmit trypanosomes and sleeping sickness throughout the entire human population in its range. Here Jamot could be successful in reaching and treating total populations since the swamps kept those living in the area from establishing villages at any distance from the river courses. Faced with the necessity of identifying those people in the villages who were afflicted with sleeping sickness and those who were healthy, Jamot the prospector, hearkening to his early training as a geologist, exhaustively sought out sleeping sickness cases. He deployed one team of doctors to make the diagnoses and a follow-up team of medical assistants to treat those suffering from the disease. This system begot the only practical control strategy possible in such an area, mobile hygiene—seeking people in need of care rather than waiting for them at a central hospital. Directed first to sleeping sickness alone, the concept was widened after Jamot's death to include a variety of diseases such as leprosy, elephantiasis, yaws, and tuberculosis.

Africa brought out the man of action in Schweitzer and some of the philosophical bent in Jamot. *"Allez-vous OPP!"* (get going!) could have been an exhortation by Jamot, the man of action, to rally his doctors, sanitary assistants, and nurses to greater effort. It was instead attributed to the philosopher, Schweitzer, driving his construction workers to get moving on building hospital quarters. "Je réveillerai la race noire" (I shall awaken the black race) could easily have been a pronouncement from Schweitzer, the missionary and the philosopher, that he would open new doors of knowledge to them. But it was Jamot who made the statement signaling his desire to wipe out sleeping sickness.

The actual practice of medicine seemed to be almost a transitory phase of Schweitzer's life, a means to an end. He kept returning to his organ playing, his studies of Bach, his writings in philosophy and in religion. At his hospital he turned more to overseeing the construction of the buildings and delegated the treatment of the sick to his younger colleagues. Sleeping sickness was but one of the many diseases with which his patients were afflicted. He did not concentrate on this particular disease, and as a consequence his impact on stamping out sleeping sickness was far less than that of Jamot, who, in fashioning a career on controlling this disease, devised important new administrative techniques which became part of government policy to implement. In later years Schweitzer reported:

The Government has taken over the fight against sleeping sickness so that our only concern now is to pass on to the "Colonial Sanitary Service" any patient in whom we suspect the disease. A large camp for these patients has been established a short distance down the river. Doctors or white assistants now visit every village in a given district and examine all the inhabitants to discover by miscroscopic tests whether germs of the disease are to be found in their blood or spinal fluid. Unfortunately at the present time this disease is increasing rather than diminishing in our region.

Schweitzer's impact was felt around the world; it stemmed from the breadth of his life and work in music, philosophy, medicine, and religion. When he died in 1965 at the age of ninety, he was buried at Lambaréné in Africa under a mahogany cross he had made himself, wreathed with purple bougainvillea. Jamot's impact was felt widely in Africa and in the medical profession. When he died in 1937 at the age of fifty-eight, he was buried in France near his home town, where a sturdy granite monument marks his grave.

Creatures of their environment, Schweitzer and Jamot, as previously pointed out, developed almost exclusively the therapeutic technique—that of killing the trypanosomes but not bothering much about the fly. Encouraged by the success of this method in the tropical forested areas, Jamot applied it in and about the plains of Ouagadougou in the area that is now Upper Volta. There he found it less successful because the human population was more mobile and spread the disease extensively into the plains, though the flies responsible for transmitting trypanosomes still adhered quite closely to the riverine areas.

In the wooded savanna and thicket areas of Tanganyika (now Tanzania) and adjoining territories, the ecologist, the environment manipulator, went all out during the twenties and thirties to burn the land, hack away at the bush, and move people about—in short, to make over vast portions of the continent of Africa to rid them of tsetse flies. In these efforts, contrasting so sharply with those bent on eradicating trypanosomes from man, the "five-star" campaigner was Charles Francis Massy Swynnerton. One of the most remarkable men—white or black—that Africa has ever known, Swynnerton spent a lifetime waging a war of harassment against the tsetse.

Born in 1877 of missionary parents assigned to India, young

Swynnerton inherited from his father, who was a senior chaplain to the Indian government, a folklorist's curiosity about local people, their legends, and their oral history. Later on this interest led him to understand well the African people in the places where he worked, their relationships and responses to their environment, the vibrancy and pulsating nature of population fluctuations among the tribes of Portuguese East Africa, of the Rhodesias, and of Tanganyika.

Swynnerton had a warm personality and charm that led people to think he might enter the diplomatic service, but his flair for field observations and his love of nature prepared him for quite different posts—one, for example, as the first game warden of Tanganyika, another as director of tsetse research and reclamation there. In these assignments he masterminded man's attempts to dominate tsetse in the wilds of East Africa.

Swynnerton became a senior school prefect and a leading light in the natural history society at Lancing College, and he had gained entry to Oxford. But his parents and relatives thought he should go to South Africa to earn the family fortune, so in 1897 at the age of nineteen he arrived in Natal. There he met Guy Marshall, a Britisher who at that time owned a general store but who later became head of the Imperial Bureau of Entomology and was knighted for his services. Swynnerton took a post as an assistant in Marshall's store. Neither man was a trader by nature; they did very poorly. Next Marshall offered Swynnerton the management of a farm in Southern Rhodesia. They fared better in farming, but neither was really a farmer. Swynnerton did plant some ceara rubber and he experimented with coffee growing and stock breeding, but his real interests already lay elsewhere.

Swynnerton rapidly became a skilled naturalist and hunter. As a naturalist he developed a special interest in butterfies and birds; he dissected the birds he shot to see what they ate. He

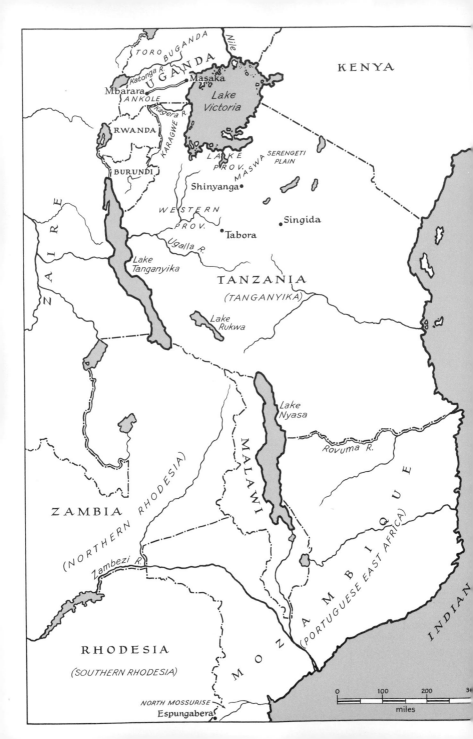

dabbed with paint the butterflies he caught so that as he found them later he could learn their patterns of flight and migration. After he had become interested in the tsetse, Swynnerton employed similar techniques to learn its habits and movements.

As a hunter, Swynnerton was not particularly sentimental about the game he shot and did not share the emotionalism of conservationists over the sometimes inevitable and even rational decimation of wildlife species. He did fear the danger of exterminating certain species through indiscriminate shooting of wildlife to eradicate tsetse. In fact, his later career centered on the search for methods other than game extermination for eliminating tsetse from East Africa. He drew up the first game laws in Tanganyika, and the advice he gave to the Uganda government led to the establishment of the Uganda Game Department.

In 1918, after a serious physical breakdown, Swynnerton left the farm and took a three-month assignment that the Mozambique Company offered him not far from his farm in southeast Rhodesia. A herd of cattle belonging to the company had suffered heavy losses from nagana near Espungabera, the official headquarters, and the company wanted to know what to do about it. He was to survey tsetse fly distribution and habits in the North Mossurise territory of Mozambique, often called Portuguese East Africa. His observations did not yield definite results but he came to two important conclusions: that properly organized settlements of human beings would be capable of clearing the country of *G. brevipalpis* and *G. pallidipes* and that annual grass fires could serve as a control for these flies if the burning were regulated and done at the proper time. The survey provided him with much basic knowledge vital to his future work.

In 1919, after World War I had ended and the British had taken over the mandated territory of Tanganyika, formerly German East Africa, the Colonial Office offered Swynnerton a post as its Director of Game Preservation. He accepted and in 1921, with the collaboration and support of Marshall, undertook tsetse fly investigations and surveys in all of the colony.

At least four species of tsetse were actively commingling and competing for space and food at this time in the prosperous mixed-farming Shinyanga District, which was named for the chiefdom that occupied the region south of Lake Victoria close to the Serengeti Plains. The species *G. palpalis,* the principal carrier of the Gambian trypanosome, clung to the river banks and bred in thickets and under rocks around the bases of many-stemmed thicket shrubs. *G. pallidipes,* Bruce's fly, like *palpalis,* loitered around the river-fringing thickets, which it used as rendevous sites for mating. *G. morsitans,* the grassland fly, was occupying the pathways and open patches of ground but not the evergreen forests or the extensive deciduous thickets. A species then unclassified but subsequently called *G. swynnertoni,* the dark brown fly with a big abdomen, was ranging over giraffe country where the tall graceful thorn trees grew.

Normally the four flies might not have attracted attention to themselves. *G. morsitans, pallidipes,* and *swynnertoni* would have continued to take their toll of cattle by transmitting to these beasts *Trypanosoma brucei,* which did not seem to infect man; *palpalis* and its *T. gambiense* that did infect man had subsided, largely because of the vigorous campaigns waged against them in Uganda early in the century. But the virulent form of sleeping sickness caused by *T. rhodesiense* had suddenly appeared and made itself felt in the Luangwa Valley of Northern Rhodesia, now Zambia, about 1910. This trypanosome was responsible in 1912 for at least seventy-seven cases of sleeping sickness along the Rovuma River, which separates Tanganyika from Mozambique. It later developed that all four of the flies, but expecially *G. morsitans,* could transmit the Rhodesian trypanosome to people.

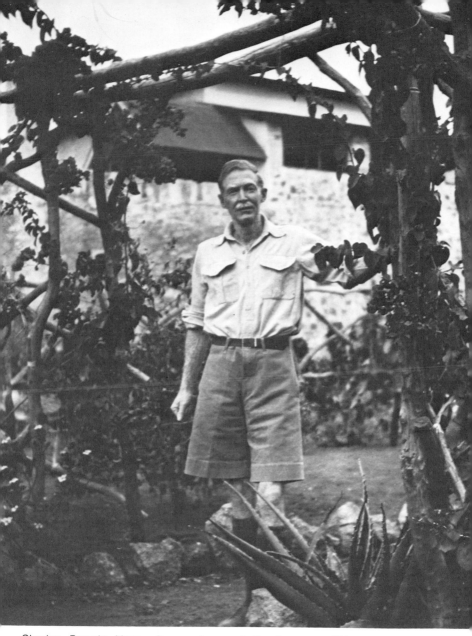

Charles Francis Massy Swynnerton and the boma at Shinyanga.
(Courtesy of R. J. M. Swynnerton.)

The headman of the town of Basheshi near Maswa in Shinyanga District reported an outbreak of disease in that area late in February 1922 and brought the matter to the attention of a Tanganyikan senior medical officer, Dr. George Maclean. The disease, first thought to be due to ancylostomiasis (hookworm), Maclean recognized as trypanosomiasis, and he at once started to build hospitals in fly-free parts of the district in order to segregate the sick.

The Maswa outbreak in the Lake Province near Lake Victoria in 1922 alarmed the governor of Tanganyika and the senior district commissioner at Tabora, Major H. C. Stiebel, as well as medical officer Maclean. It did not take long for the governor of Tanganyika on advice of his director of medical services to impress the men "round green tables" at the Colonial Office in London with the seriousness of the Maswa outbreak. They invited proposals for research and land reclamation schemes to roll back the advance of tsetse. The epidemic gave Swynnerton just the cause he needed to launch a full-scale attack against the flies. Drawing upon his observations and convictions of earlier years, he, if anyone, was prepared to blast them out of western Tanganyika. Swynnerton presented his plans to accomplish this objective late in 1922 and the Colonial Office accepted them.

Stiebel frequently went "on bivouac" with his good friend Swynnerton. He wrote:

On one occasion I was on tour with Swynnerton, and we had reached a spot five days' march from Tabora, near the Ugalla River. Our tents had been pitched about one hundred yards apart, and in the middle of the night I was awakened by what sounded like a struggle taking place in Swynnerton's tent. There was a rumbling as of a tent being violently shaken, a yell from Swynnerton, further shaking of the tent, and then silence. I shouted—there was no reply—I grabbed my shotgun and rushed to his tent. I was convinced in my own mind that a lion had got my old friend, and was wondering if I could possibly get his body back to Tabora, over a hundred miles away, or if I should bury him where we were.

I shouted again as I reached his tent—and to my relief, he replied from the bush some distance away. I met him returning to camp, dragging the hide of a Lewel Hartebeeste, which he had shot two days earlier. He calmly explained that a hyena had crept into his tent, and snatched the dry hide, which became entangled with the tent ropes. The powerful brute stuck to his prize, and nearly pulled the tent down before it got away with the hide, with Swynnerton at its heels. I spent some time endeavouring to extract a variety of thorns from my feet by the indifferent light of a paraffin lantern, and returned to my interrupted slumbers quite convinced that the collection of specimens can be overdone.

Responding to Major Stiebel's pleas, Swynnerton ultimately chose for his headquarters an abandoned German fort (*boma*) built in Shinyanga in 1912. The *boma* was not well located for research on *G. morsitans,* the main species widely distributed over the eastern part of the continent. However, it was well situated for investigations on *G. swynnertoni,* which dominated this particular area. Since the fort had hardly figured in the war, what glory it achieved came from Swynnerton's occupation of it in the fight against the fly.

The dilapidated fort was a landmark in the cruel thicket environment. In his book, *The Tsetse Flies of East Africa,* published in 1936, Swynnerton told of an old woman who customarily slept in the laboratory. Hungry, emaciated, and possibly a sleeping sickness victim, she pilfered food from the larder. She was turned outside to sleep, and one night a pack of hyenas descended upon her. She shrieked, but it was too late. Frightened eyewitnesses from the laboratory saw the hyenas one by one taking turns dragging her off a mile and a half through the bush until each had consumed its portion of the prey. The next morning, Swynnerton mixed up a strychnine bait to poison the hyenas, and from the five dead hyenas found and from the tracks and spoor of others, he estimated that at least twenty happened to be lurking around the fort.

Swynnerton thought Shinyanga District was an ideal one in which to collect firsthand information on the combination of factors that had brought about the epidemic of sleeping sickness. Before he put remedial measures into effect, he wanted to discover the relationships among game, fly, and man to such an outbreak, and he hoped to clarify their relative importance. He already had bait cattle in the field to attract flies to be captured and counted and workers plying the region to inventory the fly population.

He surveyed the Shinyanga area intensively and found three distinct types of villages that harbored sleeping sickness. The most heavily infected was the small bush village with a few isolated huts and no clearing to speak of around it. In one such village he watched the flies pester an old woman as she went about her domestic chores. A dozen or more tsetse flies rested on her leather garments and on her skin; one of Swynnerton's assistants went into her hut and captured six. Swynnerton and his crew caught approximately two hundred flies from the same village during their visit.

A village of the second type was more compact and lay at the edge of the bush; clearings bordered part of it. The tsetse fly population was less dense here than in the first type, but still three or four people had died of sleeping sickness.

A village of the third type, a rather large tribal one, occupied the center of a clearing with large millet fields surrounding it. As one would expect, still fewer tsetse flies existed here.

Swynnerton believed that the disease passed most readily from man to fly to man. Traffic and trade between villages kept sleeping sickness active in all three types, he thought. People from one village who regularly attended the sick in a neighbor-

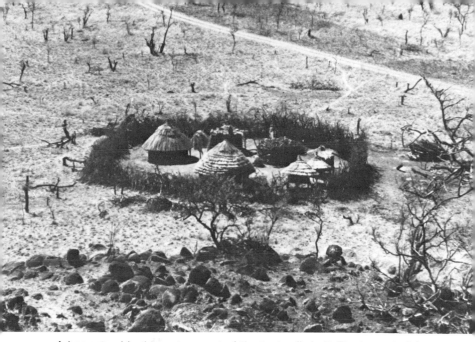

A homestead in the eastern part of the tsetse fly belt. The larger buildings are sleeping houses, the smaller ones granaries surrounded by a thorn bush hedge. (Photograph reprinted by permission from the *Geographical Review*, Vol. 50, 1960, p. 547, copyrighted by the American Geographical Society of New York.)

ing one contracted the disease and introduced it into their own village. Large social gatherings such as "beer drinks" gave tsetse flies the opportunity to pass the disease from one individual to another. Traders when they bartered for wildebeest tails contracted the disease as they passed through areas infested with tsetse flies. (The tails were important articles of commerce. Their hairs braided together gave a strong support for making bracelets, and traditional African medical practitioners prized them highly.) A man might go through an infested area to buy a hoe from a dealer in a village noted for its hoe production, perhaps staying to work in nearby salt mines to pay off the cost in labor. Women going to the water's edge exposed themselves to infection from flies that had picked up the trypanosomes from other women.

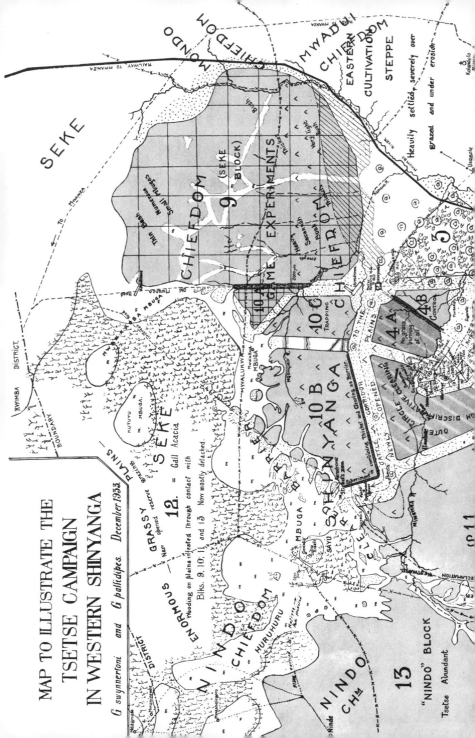

MAP TO ILLUSTRATE THE
TSETSE CAMPAIGN
IN WESTERN SHINYANGA

G. swynnertoni and *G. pallidipes.* December 1933.

ENORMOUS GRASSY PLAINS
Now opened reserve

12. = Gall Acacia

Wooding on plains invaded through contact with
Blks. 9, 10, 11 and 13. Now mostly detached.

13 "NINDO" BLOCK
Tsetse Abundant

4 A
No grass burning at all

4 B
Control

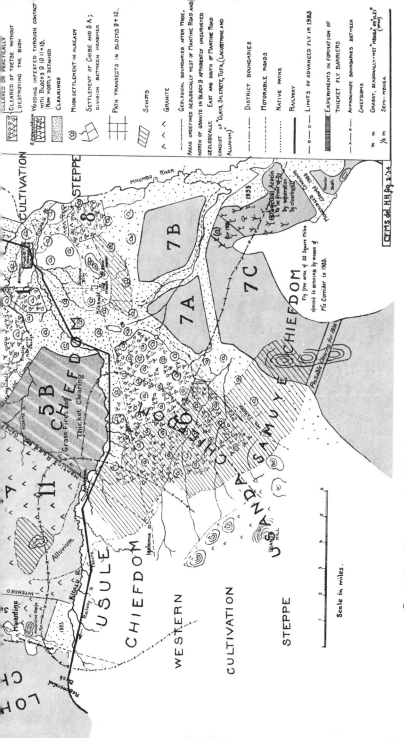

Facsimile of the map C. F. M. Swynnerton drew and used for tsetse fly experiments in Shinyanga, 1933. (*Transactions*, Vol. 84, 1936; reprinted by permission of the Royal Entomological Society of London.)

Swynnerton thought that the sleeping sickness trypanosome might also go from animals through flies to man. He therefore kept alert to countless other human activities such as collecting firewood and gathering honey, which increased man's contact with tsetse in the bush, tsetse that probably got their trypanosomes from wild animals.

The inexorable growth of the epidemic quickly led Swynnerton into grandiose research and land reclamation measures. To appreciate the scope of the research and reclamation work undertaken at Shinyanga one must refer to his *The Tsetse Flies of East Africa* and especially his freehand map charting the tsetse campaign in western Shinyanga. The map looks like one of Ernest H. Shepard's drawings marking the comings and goings of Piglet and Pooh in A. A. Milne's *Winnie the Pooh.* "Enormous grassy plains," "Nindo Chiefdom," "Weak poison experiment," "Heavy savannah bush," "Cattle corridor to the plains," and dotted trails marked "Flies carried by natives, path picketed" and other such designations decorate it. The map has a serious purpose, however, for it lays out the block system that Swynnerton and his colleagues developed for large-scale experiments of tsetse control and land reclamation. The blocks, numbering from one through thirteen, totaled nearly eight hundred square miles in area. They were of all different shapes and sizes, carved out of the bush in accordance with the topography and the vegetation and designed to fit the experiment each was destined to contain. One of the blocks, block nine, also called Seke block, was the antithesis of the pocket-handkerchief-sized plots of present-day experiments. Irregular in outline, approximately fifty square miles in area, it was intended at first for studies of the relationship of large game animals and the tsetse. Instead it came to carry the burden of exercises in the use of exclusion of fire to wipe out the fly.

Fire had been a traditional tool in the agriculture of Africa for millennia; well managed it often was a beneficial rather than a destructive one. Fires lighted early in the growing season burned away brush and dry grass to expose young shoots to livestock for feed. These small fires fed by immature grass, without much leaf litter as fuel, generated little wind to swirl the flames into the thickets and treetops to eliminate the high shade so attractive to *Glossina swynnertoni*. Large fires set in September, after the growing season, eliminated useless old brown grass. Since this was the time when grass and leaves were most abundant and driest, these late fires burned so fiercely that they sucked in a great wind. They destroyed low woody growth and many high shade-producing plants as well.

Swynnerton forged a weapon of fire by organizing the normal scattered firings during the September "late burn" season into one scheduled, collective burn directed against the tsetse. The late fires destroyed tsetse pupae and made the adult fly's life difficult by removing much of its shade, breeding places, places for concealment, and food at a hot, dry time.

For seven years beginning in 1924, Swynnerton and his scouts protected block nine against fire until late in the dry season. He fixed a date on which to fire block nine; two or three days might pass, however, before the African workers could fire the grass, for they had to wait for a favorable wind, but from the date fixed they stood posted every few hundred yards along the front awaiting the prearranged signal to ignite the grass. With luck, a fierce burn would flare up in front of a strong wind. Beyond the block those who organized fires carefully arranged simultaneous burning of contiguous fronts of land ten to twenty miles long. They tried to leave no unburned pockets that could harbor the fly.

The long walls of flames drove the tsetse before them. Many flies died of dessication or from smoke, but some became concentrated in the few places that for one reason or another did not burn. For one thing, it was hard to hold a united fire front because the front tended to break into tongues that lapped up the readily burnable areas and left some restricted places unburnt. In these concentrated pockets "fly boys"—the name given by the colonials to men and boys who caught flies and who performed a myriad of other field and laboratory tasks—hand-caught many tsetse a few days after the burns. But still substantial numbers escaped.

As the fire front advanced, grasshoppers, crickets, and other insects also flew out of their hiding places to keep ahead of it. Birds hovered over it and gorged on the disturbed insects. The line of fire flushed out rodents, snakes, small and large game; leopards and baboons, too, were ready prey to hunters. Late burning also killed ticks and other noxious insects. In Swynnerton's words, "a frequent, thorough 'burn' will be a grand general cleanser and disinfector of the country."

Sometimes the fire escaped control, burning homes and taking human lives. In his unpublished memoirs, Stiebel recalled that two men once disregarded orders not to enter the firebreak area of one of these massive burns. Days later their charred remains were found at the foot of a big tree that they evidently had climbed when they found the fire gaining on them.

Four or five good burns properly managed opened up the country. Well-burnt areas where the thickets and smaller trees were completely destroyed became incapable of supporting *swynnertoni* and other species of tsetse.

Because the savanna species of tsetse *swynnertoni* and *morsitans* liked the deep shade of thickets no better than the full light over scorched soil, Swynnerton and his colleagues also advanced quite the opposite tactic—they encouraged the growth of dense belts of impenetrable thicket by excluding the fire from areas where firing failed. They experimented with this technique over a four-square-mile area in block four and met with such success there that a few years later they put all of block nine under protection from fire, too. By 1938, seven hundred square miles of territory well beyond block nine also were under fire protection or exclusion. Here *G. swynnertoni,* at least, actually approached extinction. Some thought fire exclusion allowed fly parasites and predators to build up on tsetse; others thought that it changed air humidity and soil conditions to such an extent that it adversely affected the pupation of this insect. But no one really knew why *G. morsitans* and *G. swynnertoni* diminished so markedly when fire was excluded.

Certain patches of land which would not burn did not even lend themselves to the fire exclusion technique. Heavy clay and hard-pan soil, for instance, would not sustain the growth of enough thicket to support a good burn, much less qualify for fire exclusion. For these and some other areas, Swynnerton tried a progressive annual demolition of the fly "belt" by clear ing the growth it did carry with pangas, long broad-bladed knives similar to the South American machete. Bush was rapidly encroaching on good cattle country, and the related advance of the fly was leaving extremely inadequate areas for grazing. In one chiefdom alone over a period of years the population shrank from 30,000 persons to little more than 5,000. There was an urgent need to reverse this trend.

The chiefs knew that one really effective way to stop bush and fly encroachment was to hack away the bush each year on the margin of their grazing land. Because each chiefdom was law unto itself and no one chiefdom exerted power over another, mobilizing the people of several contiguous chiefdoms to work together called for direction of a central authority—in this case, the colonial administration.

In November of 1923 the colonial administrative officer for the Shinyanga District arranged a meeting of the chiefs of the area. Swynnerton attended it; he told them that they had the weapons, pangas, for fly exterminations in their own hands. So he encouraged them to slash the bush, using their pangas in a large experimental area.

The experimental annual clearing project got under way in May 1924. Swynnerton chose as his lieutenants people from all walks of life in the natural sciences: B. D. Burtt, a botanist; John F. V. Phillips, an ecologist; W. H. Potts, C. H. N. Jackson, and T. A. M. Nash, entomologists; G. St. Clair Thompson, a forester who also served as curator and librarian; and S. P. Teare, a game warden.

In the massive bush-clearing campaign, Swynnerton directed the people and supervised the work personally, giving due regard to the nature and the amount of bush to be cleared along the front and to the population of each chiefdom. Four chiefdoms furnished 2,000 men, four supplied 4,500, and two others sent out 1,400 men to clear at the bush margins of their adjoining areas. Blacksmiths and men who fashioned wooden handles shaped and repaired the cutting tools. As the campaign progressed, some workers tired and left; others rallied to the cause. In all, more than 10,000 men engaged in the operation during the first season. The chiefs exhorted their people to action. They described tsetse as the enemy, the workers as soldiers in battle. Clearing included dragging, piling, and burning of the felled trees. Not content with marginal clearing of the youngest bush only, the people frequently cleared solid blocks of land, thereby reclaiming at once a worthwhile grazing space. Swynnerton later reported that people responded to encouragement, they worked with a will, sang at their work, and in several of the camps danced every night.

Thousands of people clearing the land by fire or sword might advance indefinitely into tsetse-infested bush, searing new ground, leaving vast "cleansed" and cleared areas behind that might grow into bushland again but free from the fly. But scarcity of people to settle and to develop the reclaimed land turned out to be the greatest handicap to the success of these antitsetse measures. Areas with population as low as one person per square mile could not sustain an epidemic of sleeping sickness. Twenty-five persons per square mile provided a population density sufficient to clear land of bush so that the people could till it and thereby reduce the fly population; it also constituted a population sufficiently dense to maintain an epidemic. A hundred persons per square mile automatically produced fly-free areas cleared and cropped—a "no fly's land" surrounding and protecting them from the carrier of sleeping sickness and thus sleeping sickness itself.

Swynnerton's efforts notwithstanding, the Rhodesian disease first recognized at Maswa seemed to be spreading and gaining ground. It had burst into a devastating epidemic near Lake Rukwa farther south, and by 1930 it involved all of the Western Province and part of the Lake Province where Shinyanga was located. By 1929 more than 3,000 cases were reported, over 2,000 from one district alone.

Measures to establish or reestablish large compact population centers were viewed as essential either to make use of land already cleared or to develop new tsetse-free pockets in uncleared bush country. These measures heralded another grand-scale attack—to pit the population density of human beings, as though masses of people were a weapon, against that of the fly. To do this, governmental authorities had to locate the taxpayers in the stricken area and from them construct a population census to gain some notion of the resettlement problem at hand. They also had to discuss probable new village sites to which these people could move. A sleeping sickness surveyor, accompanied by several tribal elders, surveyed the district for such sites and helped to choose suitable cropland in parcels as nearly square as possible, about sixteen acres for each family. In one

case in 1936, people of a tribal group numbering 1,251 taxpayers but having a total population of 3,353 were moved an average distance of twenty miles. To transport this group in its entirety took fifty-one days; trucks clocked a total of 22,149 miles
to carry these people and their belongings. But the expense of
moving the entire village came to less than £500, an average
cost per person of three shillings and two pence.

Resettling such people was a complicated process. Those in
need of resettling normally lived at a bare subsistence level.
Some had to be provided employment, others taught how to
produce food and cash crops on newly acquired land, still others to be reintroduced to cattle husbandry, for they had long
ago lost the art of keeping cattle.

Many people resented being drawn away from their bush villages. If they could not live where they were born, at least they
wished to go home to die, and they kept filtering back to their
old homesites.

Rallying the people 5,000 to 10,000 at a time to fire or
clear the land and reorganizing villages were "wholesale" control measures that became more difficult and costly to implement year after year. Insects other than tsetse also competed for
man's time and attention. Sometimes locusts built up to plague
proportions around Shinyanga. Naturally, when they swarmed
over an area, the local tsetse control forces would abandon
tsetse control measures and organize to keep the locusts off of
their crops.

Daring action requisite for "wholesale" fly eradication had to
be tempered by sophisticated and subtle attacks that depended
upon precision techniques. The subtle approach, akin to sniping
at the enemy, demanded an increasingly thorough knowledge of
the association of the fly with its environment—where it was
weakest, where it was most tenacious, what species of plants
harbored it most successfully. One of the most important of the

precision techniques was discriminative clearing. This technique depended on carefully selecting the area to be cleared and on subtracting from the environment only those plants in any given area that tsetse absolutely could not do without.

Precision techniques also evoked imagination and ingenuity. Poisons to kill brush were too expensive to apply. Swynnerton's deputy director, Dr. John Phillips the ecologist, had applied arsenic pentoxide and sodium chlorate in auger holes which he bored in the trunks and in "frills" cut around the boles of the trees; but the arsenicals were toxic and only partially effective, the sodium chlorate too expensive. In one area thick with tsetse flies and in need of clearing, the big trees and the heavy brush were too hard to cut with pangas. There were no bulldozers in East Africa at that time, not until after World War II. There was, in fact, no mechanized equipment of any kind in that area in the 1920's and 1930's. Why not let the termites fell the trees? Swynnerton's scouts did just that. Where clearing was imperative, they girdled the bark of the large trees, piled dirt around the trunks, and waited for the termites to rise up from the soil, attack, and rot out the heart of the trees, which then became "pushovers."

Game destruction, another "wholesale" measure, had for years been part of Swynnerton's master plan of tsetse fly control. But it was his followers, rather than Swynnerton himself, who carried out the game destruction experiment, the one for which he had originally laid out block nine. In 1938, in the course of a routine aerial survey of game movements, Swynnerton and his botanist colleague, Burtt, skimmed over the bush at too low an altitude. The plane crashed near Singida and closed both their careers.

In 1948, ten years after his death, Swynnerton's former lieutenants annexed to the already extensive experimental land at Shinyanga four additional blocks—thirteen through sixteen. All told, this new area measured more than six hundred square miles; it supported a game population of ten animals per square mile. They set up these blocks to try to answer the question Swynnerton had posed in earlier years—would destroying all big game really eliminate the fly? And if the larger game were gone could the flies survive on the smaller game, such as pigs and small antelope like duiker? But the game population was not static. During the five-year period of the experiment, animals moved in and out. Village settlements bounded three of the four sides of the newly acquired blocks. The fourth side, fifty miles long, was open to game and the bush. The Shinyanga workers constructed a five-strand barbed-wire fence along this side in an attempt to prevent reentry of game. Still, to exhaust the area of big game, hunters had to shoot more than eight thousand rhinoceros, giraffe, lion, antelope, and gazelle. In doing so, they left the savanna species of tsetse in the area— *swynnertoni, morsitans,* and *pallidipes*—a hungry community of flies on a starvation diet.

The experiment was a great success: *G. swynnertoni* and *G. morsitans* disappeared completely; *G. pallidipes* hung on in exceedingly small numbers. The cost for the initial extermination of the game animals amounted to fifty pounds per square mile —cheaper than firing, excluding fire, or clearing land, but what good was the area with the game gone? Those who managed the exercise recommended at its termination that other methods of control be put into effect, not really out of regard for game animals but rather because other measures proved more practical and, in the end, even more economical.

Finally the epidemic of sleeping sickness ran its course, but not without taking a substantial toll of human life. Between 1922 and 1946, 23,000 people were diagnosed as having sleeping sickness in Tanganyika. In 1948 the territory's Sleeping Sickness Officer, Dr. H. Fairbairn, estimated that at a cure rate of about 48 per cent, which was recorded for Tabora in Western Province, a minimum of 11,500 either had died or would die. And the fly still prevailed.

Spectacular and drastic as some of the immediate massive control measures were, ingenious as discriminative and selective ones appeared to be, permanent control of sleeping sickness and nagana in eastern Africa seemed to the colonial experts to depend upon what people did with the land freed of tsetse and what population density they themselves maintained in these areas. Often their ideas of village organization and of land use seemed to foster rather than depress tsetse populations or to damage their environment in other ways. It is interesting to note that one governor of Tanganyika, Sir Donald Cameron, was not always in sympathy with Swynnerton's approach, and in October 1928 Dr. Phillips, Swynnerton's colleague, went to Cameron to intercede for his chief about finances for the next five years. In response to Cameron's question, "If I greatly augment the amount of support for Tsetse work, would you, within a given time, clear Tsetse fly from certain areas of Tanganyika?" Phillips replied: "If I could, I wouldn't because this Government, like every other Government in Africa, is not prepared to apply *livestock control*—the result of opening up country against the Tsetse fly in the absence of livestock culling and management would mean the coming in of a greater curse than Tsetse, deterioration and erosion!"

Twenty-one years later, 1949, the same man, Phillips, took the same stand with the governor of the time, Sir Edward Twining, in the same room, in front of the same map of Tanganyika as in October 1928, and the governor remarked with a twinkle in his eye: "We are no more ready today to do what you said to Cameron twenty years ago, and the result is that it is still stalemate; *there is more fly today than there was twenty years ago in Tanganyika!*" (Italics added in both quotations.)

Swynnerton's methods and his programs—for example, discriminative clearing and pitting human population pressures against those of the fly—had a wide and lasting impact on tsetse fly control and eradication programs in Africa. An example is the later work of Dr. T. A. M. Nash, one of Swynnerton's colleagues, a medical entomologist who carried the battle of the fly to Nigeria in West Africa, where he used some of the same basic techniques as did Swynnerton in his sparkling campaign in East Africa.

Nash emphasized resettling people and rural development so that the people would have a means for earning a living in the area he carved out of bush and freed of tsetse flies for them. So far did Nash go in organizing villages free of fly and of disease that he created virtually antiseptic hamlets, which for reasons quite different from fear of contracting sleeping sickness proved to be beyond the will of the masses of people to maintain.

When the dust from the Sahara harmattan winds blots out the sun, one can close his eyes and sniff his way through Kano, a not-exactly-antiseptic city in northern Nigeria, but a city similar to many others in the world. Dung smells announce the outskirts of Kano, where the animals glean sorghum and millet stubble from the sun-baked fields. Night soil and sewage odors identify the gardens of lettuce and onions, growing along the intermittent streams in the "suburbs" of the city. The smell of burnt animal hair, flesh, and bone from the abattoirs and tanneries marks the industrial sections. A faint aroma of peanut butter or of peanut brittle cooking suggests nearness to the groundnut (peanut) processing plants and to the pyramids of nuts waiting to be shipped abroad or to be crushed for oil. In the European section, the neem tree, an import from India, laden with yellow flowers, spreads its pungent and somewhat oppressive perfume along the broad avenues.

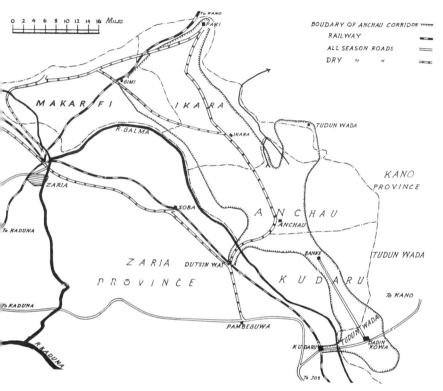

The Anchau Corridor. (Drawing from T. A. M. Nash, *The Anchau Rural Development and Settlement Scheme*, London, 1948. British Crown copyright; by permission of the Controller of Her Britannic Majesty's Stationery Office.)

Fifty-five miles south of Kano lies the Anchau Corridor, which is an arbitrarily delineated strip of land along a watershed which cuts through a number of adjacent political districts and covers 712 square miles. Today Anchau Corridor looks like many other parts of northern Nigeria and the rest of the rural world. The soil, where exposed, has a reddish-brown hue. The roadways through the area are rutty and unkempt. Low places support scrub trees and thicket bushes; the high areas in some zones display fine grass six to eight feet tall; in other places there are concentrated farming operations—patchy fields of cotton, tobacco, groundnuts, maize, and sorghum, which in Africa, where it originated, is called Guinea corn. Swampy depressions where sugarcane breaks out in massive waves of feathery tassels interrupt the monotony of the corridor, which is relatively flat. The Galma River, but a trickle at the close of the dry season, runs southwest of the corridor in a sweeping, shallow valley. On the banks of this once tsetse-infested river and its tributaries and on the high points above the marshy areas people crowd into compact villages of round houses with thatched roofs. About fifty thousand Hausa people made their homes there in scattered villages when the corridor's formation was proposed in 1936 as a means of organizing people in an area that could be made and kept free of tsetse. Nomadic Fulani, the traditional cattle herders, intermingled with the sedentary Hausas. The shape of the corridor was important and it was designed to link the fly-free area of one district with those of others, so that people could go from one clear area to another without having to pass through fly-infested ones.

In 1933 the district of Anchau and its headquarters, old Anchau, as well as neighboring districts making up the corridor, were suffering from a full-blown epidemic of sleeping sickness. As in Uganda thirty years earlier, a third of the population of these Nigerian villages had sleeping sickness; in some hamlets half the population was affected.

Nash, a medical entomologist, set out to change all this. His mandate to attack the epidemic grew out of an entirely relevant question Dr. Walter Johnson, director of medical services in Nigeria, had asked Nash when he visited Swynnerton's Shinyanga project in the late 1920's. The question was, how could one keep horses in the heart of a fly belt in Nigeria? Although his main consideration was to control sleeping sickness in man, still it was a matter of personal as well as administrative concern to Johnson, a keen horseman, to be able to ride through fly belts. As it was, Johnson, with bicycle strapped to his back, forded many a stream, all the parasitic diseases the water carried notwithstanding. Nash was down with dysentery and therefore not in his best form when he and Johnson first met in Shinyanga. Nevertheless, Johnson later wrote Nash a personal letter inviting him to Nigeria to investigate trypanosomiasis in man and livestock. Nash decided to go and spent seven years carrying the chief responsibility for eliminating sleeping sickness in Anchau.

Nash made a preliminary survey of the area destined to become Anchau Corridor. He found that the population, largely Hausa, had fanned out to many small but congested villages along tsetse-infested streams. These villages lacked sufficient clearing around them to insulate them from the fly. Much of the area between the villages was so sparsely settled that tsetse from the riverine vegetation readily dominated both bush and village. When the people went out in search of water and fuel they were easy prey for the fly; in the villages the fly spread sleeping sickness easily from one person to another. Nash felt that it would be necessary to reorganize the villages to achieve a population level of seventy people per square mile, which he regarded as the minimum for maintaining the stream banks free of tsetse after the initial clearing to eliminate the fly.

The corridor had practical features which favored fly control and rural development. Its network of communications was good. The Zaria-Kano railroad bordered it in the north and the Zaria-Jos Railroad line ran along its southwestern side. A dry-season road cut through its center, and it was served by an all-season road to the south. Such was the intensity of the fly population and the incidence of sleeping sickness that the results of a campaign to eliminate the fly and stamp out the disease could easily be measured.

Previous research had shown the tsetse species *G. tachinoides* to be eradicable by discriminative clearing; it was the principal carrier of sleeping sickness and it infested most of the area. Its companion *G. palpalis,* which is more difficult to control, occupied only the southern part of the district, and it was hoped that the clearing techniques would create low-humidity areas there that would be unacceptable for it, too.

G. tachinoides, at the northern limit of its range, was confined for breeding and resting sites mainly to the thickets and bushes of the rivers and streams. Like people who built their villages near a source of water, the fly had to have moisture. Nash therefore recommended the removal of the undergrowth and low branching trees from these fly habitats. This method, which he called partial clearing, was similar to discriminative clearing so successfully used in East Africa to gain areas free of the woodland fly. Nash also recommended resettlement of the people in such areas. On his advice, Johnson (now Sir Walter) and his colleague, Dr. H. M. O. Lester, drafted a scheme using these two means for eradicating tsetse from the Anchau Corridor. Before approving the project in 1936, the Colonial Office wisely advised that economic development must form an essential part of the plan. The Sleeping Sickness Service of Nigeria assumed responsibility for implementing the scheme. In the short run it turned out to be an amazingly successful venture in rural development and settlement—the first of its kind in West Africa. The cost for all works connected with the program during the ten-year period it was pursued inside and outside the corridor came to £85,000, between one and two pounds per person involved.

As Sir Hesketh Bell in Uganda and Swynnerton in Tanzania had stressed in their campaigns, Nash, too, emphasized the importance of breaking the "togetherness" which nature imposed on man and fly. In Anchau this meant opening up the stream banks to sunlight and to hot, dry winds. The fly would have nowhere else to go; it could not survive along the cutover areas.

Shady groves by the water's edge offered a common meeting ground for man and fly. This was a biting truth in one of the small Nigerian hamlets in the corridor housing forty-three people, thirty of whom had sleeping sickness. This hamlet dominated a small stream that dried up after the rains. During the dry season, not a pool of water nor a single tsetse could be found for miles up and down the stream bed. Close to the hamlet, however, the sand in the bed was moist. Here villagers had scooped out a hole two feet deep to enable water to collect. Each woman from the village took her turn sitting by the hole. She would scrape up a cupful of water with a curved section of a calabash, transfer it to her water jug, then wait for water to seep into the hole again. It took each woman about fifteen minutes to fill her jug. Nash, watching the process for hours, caught only four specimens of tsetse, but though the numbers were small here he concluded that the man-fly contact was extremely intense. He estimated that fewer than a dozen tsetse flies fed on a queue of women for many hours each day, inoculating many with disease, and in the process expending minimal energy in the search for food.

As at Shinyanga in Tanzania, so in Anchau in Nigeria the clearing technique required a massive labor force. If three hundred men were employed to clear a stream, they might be divided into three gangs—an advance gang of 75 panga men, a center gang of 75 ax men, and a rear guard of 150 pilers. The men with the pangas started to clear the undergrowth; then the second gang chosen for their physique and armed with heavy axes came along to cut down the low-branched shade trees. They roped the trees that leaned over the stream. When these trees were ready to fall, the men pulled them so they would crash upon the banks. The piling gang followed the ax men and dragged the brush over to the tree stumps, where they built bonfires. To keep up with the men cutting undergrowth and shade trees, this gang had to be double the size of the others. One European, Nash later reported, could direct six hundred laborers working on two or three different streams; such an aggregation could clear up to forty-five miles of stream bank in two months. The clearings were always started at the stream sources so as to push the fly downstream and out of the corridor. Cost of the heavy initial clearing was paid for at then current rates; unpaid community labor, which was recruited under the provisions of the 1937 Sleeping Sickness Ordinance, accomplished almost all of the subsequent slashing and reslashing of regrowth over the years.

Nash and his colleagues adhered to the system of indirect rule which Lord Lugard had established in northern Nigeria in the early 1900's. This meant that the local government, which was called Native Authority, and the colonial government each had its special responsibility and authority. The draft for local labor came through the Native Authority. If the labor turnout proved disappointingly low, the top Nigerian leader of the province, the emir, sometimes had to be persuaded to bring pressure on the village chieftain to get the clearing done. Usually, reslashing required three to four days' work per man per year. It took seven years for the most persistent stumps to die out, but by that time almost all regrowth of stump sprouts ceased.

Not always did it prove wise to clear the stream banks in the Anchau region. For example, the value of the raffia palm, which grew along many of the streams, had to be considered.

Pole cutters in the area sought the mid-ribs of the palm fronds for use as long, straight, light poles for rafters to support thatched roofs. No other material in the area served as well for this purpose. But the raffia palm also afforded excellent harboring sites for *G. tachinoides,* and the pole cutters working in the groves unavoidably exposed themselves to the fly. Naturally, the incidence of sleeping sickness was high among them.

Nash might have recommended clearing the stream banks choked with raffia palm, but then he would have ruined this important industry. Instead he introduced a system which limited the cutters' entrance to the groves to periods when the tsetse flies could not infect them. In a protected place, a thatched hut, for example, male flies lived as long as ninety-three days, females as long as 116 days. The mean life span was less than fifty days. Under field conditions where predators and shortages of food took their toll, sixty-nine days was the greatest period of longevity recorded. Seventy-five days became an arbitrary choice for the probable maximum longevity of flies in the heart of the raffia palm groves. The incubation period for trypanosomes in flies was eighteen days; during that period a fly's bite could not infect man. Under Nash's plan, which assumes neglible migration of infected flies from other areas, pole cutters could enter the groves only during the first fourteen days of each quarter of the year. They could stay no longer, for if one pole cutter entered the area with transmissible parasites in his blood the tsetse flies would pick them up and eighteen days later be able to transmit them to another pole cutter. Seventy-five days had to elapse before the next cutting period so that almost all individuals of the generation of the flies infected by any man who had parasites in his blood would be dead. A new, "clean" batch of flies would have taken their place.

The men in the bush seemed at least partially prepared to accept manipulations of their environment like partial clearing, especially if these manipulations fit well with their ideas about how they could prosper. Planting sugarcane had become profitable; in the low marshy areas, this fact more than fear of disease prompted the local dwellers to clear the marshes and free them of flies. These same men were far less ready to accept reshuffling of their villages—to them an extremely difficult social adjustment the reason for which they could not understand. Consequently, carrying out what they saw as a necessity for resettlement taxed the ingenuity of Nash and his colleagues much more than did partial clearing.

To destroy some villages, to move others, and to create new ones, Nash needed an intensive analysis of the physical characteristics of the corridor and a thorough understanding of the life of the people. Therefore his team identified and mapped all the streams, tributaries, native wells, paths, trade routes, and villages. They put milestones on all roads and trade routes.

Existing population density and future family expansion came under review. The leaders of the scheme ran a census and determined the village areas to which the hamlets belonged so as to be sure that the villages, when moved, would remain under the control of their own headmen. Next they studied family size in the hamlets, the amount of land each farmer tilled close to his house, how he farmed it, and what outlying farms he operated. The team investigated water and fuel consumption per capita. Nash and his colleagues also had to find out what sort of bush land would make good farmland. They relied upon the local plants, some of which grew on poor soil, others on good soil only, to tell them where the soil was adequate for farming and where it was not; and they sought possible sources of water.

Overseers and surveyors alike were deeply involved in the field operations. Nash studied Hausa, a language not easy to learn with its different dialects; it took him three or four years to master it.

In a few cases, those directing the scheme made mistakes. In one instance they recommended that the people move their village to high, fly-free ground; the people complied. This site proved, for inexplicable reasons, to be damp. When the water table rose unduly after the rains, the floors and the walls of the new houses absorbed the water and the mud walls dissolved.

Nash and his colleagues also met with stubborn resistance to their recommendations. One could expect no less. Emir or headman ordered the people to move to tsetse-free areas; they were expected to obey such orders, although they usually did not understand the reasons. All the subtleties of the disease, including its long incubation period, its constant presence, and its sneaky mode of contact, were difficult to grasp, and so those living in the corridor were usually ignorant and hence apathetic about the harm it was really inflicting on them.

The Kudumi people refused to move to a tsetse-free area for what they considered very good reasons. They had valuable sugarcane farms where they were, and living as they did, miles away from anyone else, they had built a lucrative business harboring thieves from the Kano emirate who used their village as a refuge. The Kudumi people fled to Kano rather than move to the new village site. But they fared poorly in Kano, then reconsidered, and finally settled in the village prepared for them. They soon became one of the most prosperous and content of the resettled peoples in the corridor.

Deep in the corridor lay provincial old Anchau, which, when the scheme began, was far less antiseptic than cosmopolitan Kano is today. Nash found old Anchau and other cities "indescribably filthy." He wrote about old Anchau:

Some 2,500 people lived within a town wall which surrounded only 0.118 of a square mile, giving a population density rate of 21,200 to the square mile; on the weekly market day about 3,000 additional people would crowd into it—a seething mob, all coughing, sneezing, and spitting, owing to irritation from the peppers which were on sale in most of the tumble-down little booths. Any diseases in the town were readily spread to the villages after market days. The town was traversed by sunken foot-paths, winding between high mat fences, and ankle deep in spat-out sugarcane fibre; wooden clogs were worn in the rains because of the mud. Stinking borrow pits and dye pits mingled their smells with the all-prevailing odour of human excrement, which was voided round the town wall and in the few open spaces. For defensive reasons the town had been built on the edge of a marsh, with two tsetse-infested streams on the west and south; in addition, tsetse swarmed in the thicket-choked moat of the town wall, which the people objected to clearing because, according to prophecy, its removal would lead to the destruction of the town; the thicket was cleared, but Anchau survives. Mosquitoes came up at dusk from the marsh and borrow pits in countless myriads. For years all beasts had been slaughtered on a piece of blood-soaked ground, littered with paunch contents and bones, and providing a meeting-place for the hyaena and vulture populations. The dead were buried inside the town in hopes that the hyaenas would not find them. In the wet season, guinea corn, growing fourteen feet in height, would choke the few open spaces. Water was obtained from the swamp or from filthy wells, often sited within a few yards of a pit latrine. Such was Anchau, the district headquarters.

Old Anchau, steeped in tradition and a symbol of the political life of the district, could not be moved—but it might be improved. Amid wide-open spaces, it had become, in Nash's view, a slum city, ripe for slum clearance and urban renewal. But even to start to improve old Anchau required moving people out of the town, and this in turn necessitated building a new town a mile away. So in 1939 Nash's men assisted the district officer in creating an antiseptic city called Takalafiya, meaning "walk in health," a mile west of old Anchau, to siphon off some of the excess population from the old town and open up possibilities for renovating it.

Plan of old Anchau. (Drawing from Nash; British Crown copyright; by permiss the Controller of Her Britannic Majesty's Stationery Office.)

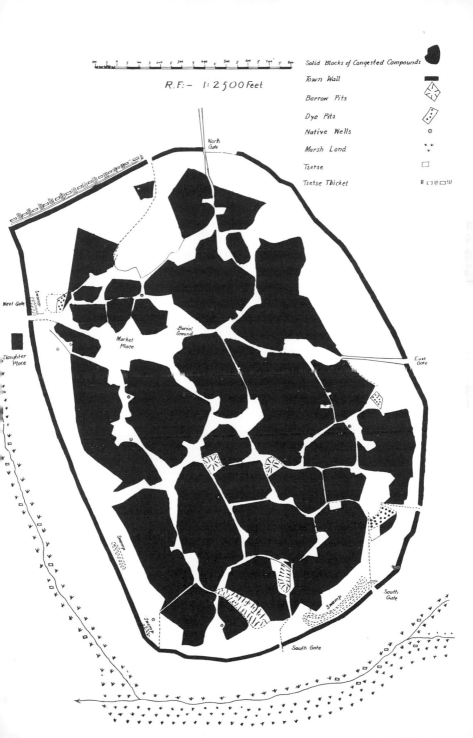

R.F:- 1:2500 Feet

Solid Blocks of Congested Compounds
Town Wall
Borrow Pits
Dye Pits
Native Wells
Marsh Land
Tsetse
Tsetse Thicket

North Gate

West Gate

Swamp

Slaughter Place

Market Place

Burial Ground

East Gate

Swamp

Swamp

Swamp

Swamp

South Gate

South Gate

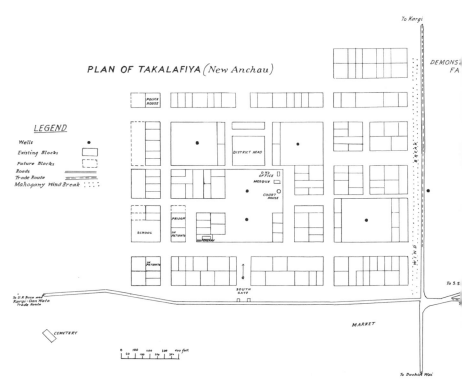

Plan of Takalafiya. (Drawing from Nash; British Crown copyright; by permission of the Controller of Her Britannic Majesty's Stationery Office.)

"The townsmen from old Anchau . . . proved far more intractable than the peasants" who lived in small villages and hamlets. Anchau residents had, according to Nash, "the typical, but understandable, slum dwellers' mentality," a culture of poverty. Nevertheless he and his men persuaded six hundred people, nearly a fourth of the population, to move from old Anchau to Takalafiya. In 1943, 270 more people joined the six hundred, and by 1948 the population stood at well over one thousand, including Native Administration officials and government employees.

The same innovations carried out in the villages were used in Takalafiya. These included introducing drains and planting as live fences oil of ben trees, whose leaves, rich in vitamins, were used in soups. The city folk were encouraged to plant trees bearing fruit that would give them a more varied and nutritious diet. All roadways were made one hundred feet wide, partly to act as firebreaks. They were lined with mahogany, mango, fig, and yellow-flowered cassia trees. The new city included a stone dispensary, an elementary school, a mosque, a courthouse and a prison. Nash and his group encouraged the local weaving industry and trading in beeswax, silk, and many other commodities.

A modern market was built with permanent stalls that contrasted sharply with the flimsy shacks of the market in old Anchau.

But a market had to "take." It was not something foreigners could readily establish even if they had the best intentions in the world and took great care to consult the local people. To assure the market's success, the residents had to "collect all the spirits and . . . attend to their affairs." This implied bringing gifts to them, as a Hausa woman, Baba of Karo, pointed out in her description of a similar situation, the move from Old Giwa to New Giwa—but when New Giwa was built, not even overtime work of the *Bori* (spirit) dancers availed to assure the economic vitality of this market.

After the removal of the first six hundred people from old Anchau and construction of the new market in Takalafiya, it then became possible to clean up old Anchau—to cut a roadway one hundred feet wide down the length of the city and two fifty-foot passages across it. This did much to relieve congestion and to dissipate the smells. But "There is no smell of cattle dung. It is like a hospital. A town must have the smell of cattle to please a Fulani," wrote the Nigerian novelist Cyprian Ekwensi of New Chanka in his novel *Burning Grass*. Surely some of the smells in old Anchau must have been essential to please the Hausas. Every town and village must have its own characteristic smells.

The old huts were broken up and thrown into the mud pits which were used to dig for adobe. The dumps were planted to eucalyptus trees, which took up much of the stagnant water that the pits held, and water remained in them for a few weeks of the year only, instead of for months as it had before. Drains were cut to keep the moat around the town wall dry. Abandoned dye pits with their wriggling mosquito larvae were filled in, as were the contaminated wells. Five modern wells were dug.

Improved old Anchau and modern, antiseptic Takalafiya had a great immediate impact. Sleeping sickness disappeared, the general health and vitality of the people improved. Having eradicated the disease and the fly in the corridor, having upgraded village life, and having renovated old Anchau and built Takalafiya, the Sleeping Sickness Service relinquished control of these towns and, in fact, the entire corridor to the local Native Administration by 1949.

One of Nash's assistants in Nigeria was Alhaji (short for "I have made a pilgrimage to Mecca") Da'u, who has since risen to the position of senior field officer with the Nigerian Institute for Trypanosomiasis Research. Advancing from a wage of four pence a day to a salary of four hundred pounds a year, Alhaji Da'u is an outstanding example of a successful "fly boy."

Under his guidance fifty men with the titles of field assistants, research assistants, laboratory assistants, and technical assistants do the work once done by those called simply "fly boys." With firm chin and lips and wispy goatee, and with an

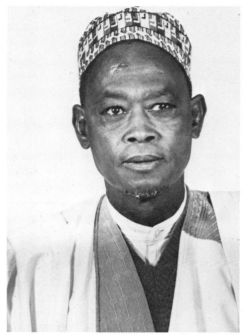

Alhaji Da'u. (Photograph supplied by Dr. T. M. Leach.)

innate dignity strengthened by years of experience working in two cultures, he combines the costumes of each as is customary among his people. When I met him he wore a white pillbox type of hat with a varicolored checkered border, a flowing yellow *riga* Nigerian style over a brown business suit, a white crocheted scarf, and sandals. Over sixty, coughing frequently— probably from long exposure to dust during his rugged years in the bush—he is near the close of his career.

When reviewing his labors at the Anchau Rural Development and Settlement Scheme, Alhaji Da'u complained sadly that the people later abandoned the important innovations he tried to get them to accept to protect themselves from tsetse attack. Yet when asked whether these efforts were worth it, he said without hesitation, "Yes, they were," and that he would again embark upon a rural development effort based on eradicating tsetse from an area if he had the opportunity to do so.

In 1967, I visited Takalafiya and the remodeled old Anchau with Alhaji Da'u. Neither city appeared to have remained permanently antiseptic. A generation after its creation as a city of health, Takalafiya looked about like old Anchau; both cities resembled old Anchau as Nash had described it in the late 1930's, just as the Anchau scheme got under way. The market "took" in Takalafiya evidently, for in the marketplace a variety of small stalls with artistic, twisted poles propping up thatched roofs filled the spaces between the model vending shelters supported by straight cement posts, now in disrepair. Tobacco, maize, and garden crops had gradually crept over the broad playgrounds with central wells that Nash and his team had provided to prevent contamination from pit latrines and to provide firebreaks. No new wells replaced the old ones dug twenty-seven to thirty years ago. The old wells were not repaired; their pulleys, iron fittings, and ropes had long since disappeared. As of old, the people drew water from the wells with their own ropes and collapsible goatskin buckets.

The pathway from the town to the slaughter slab was overgrown with weeds, and the slab itself looked infrequently used. The crumbling cement showed that it had certainly never been resurfaced. The mango and other fruit trees were old and ragged; no new trees supplemented them. Huts built along traditional lines filled the thirteen-yard spaces between houses, the minimum zoning allotment recommended in the compounds. The streets had fallen into such a state of disrepair that it was out of the question for a car or even a jeep to use them. Many small children, plagued with drippy noses, crowded the compounds and the streets.

The medical dispensary was also in disrepair. The registry

for recording the prevailing diseases of the townspeople was unintelligible and obviously used for purposes other than to tabulate health statistics in an organized fashion. Alhaji Da'u decided to write in the registry as one would write in a guest book, to let the villagers know that after an absence of four or five years he had passed through the town again. He groped for a pen among those that the dispensary assistant offered him. All that were available were broken ballpoint pens—none of them in condition for writing. On the veranda of the dispensary slouched a middle-aged man, recovering from wounds probably inflicted in a panga fight. Great gobs of purple ointment were spread over his arms and legs as salve for his wounds, and he smelled of carbolic acid.

A new generation occupied, overcrowded the once-model city of Takalafiya. Urban renewal amid wide-open spaces seemed to me once again to be a crucial need. Sleeping sickness and the fly had yet to return, either to Takalafiya or to old Anchau, but given time they surely would.

The resounding success in Anchau belonged to a by-gone generation and to a foreign culture; it did not "take" sufficiently to become an integral part of the lives of a new generation. Relieved of the pressure of an epidemic, who wanted to live in a hospital (Takalafiya) instead of a home (old Anchau)? Objectives other than sleeping sickness control, rural transformation, and village improvement according to western standards were important to people. Time still was required. Education of the masses in a western sense and to western values, if they wished it, had to take place and local leadership toward these goals had to develop before the elements of disease control and of rural development once imposed on the people from abroad could or would become a natural part of their lives.

A great army of African workers burgeoned in field, laboratory, and office as the campaigns against tsetse progressed.

These workers made it possible for Nash, Swynnerton, and others to succeed in the battles against the fly. They walked miles in the field to catch flies, to set fly traps, and to survey tsetse populations; and they performed expertly a variety of assignments in the laboratories. Many of them, whether men or young boys, built lifetime careers as "fly boys," a respected title in its heyday—one which has given way to the more appropriate designations field assistant, technician, tsetse fly officer, and the like. The labor-intensive tactics central to the execution of the campaigns depended upon these workers; leadership often arose from their midst.

Swedi Abdallah, for one, became an outstanding "noncommissioned officer" of the great African labor force in Swynnerton's campaign of the 1920's. Decades later Nash in conversation recalled Swedi as "a wonderful old character, with huge feet and a frightful stammer," a great naturalist who knew all trees, plants, animals, and their tracks. Swedi's energy was boundless and his knowledge of the various tsetses great. In 1922 he ferreted out sleeping sickness victims who in those days were frequently hidden by relatives. Once, threatened by spearmen, he meekly accompanied them as a hostage as far as their chief and there won his release. Another time he followed a difficult case in which the relatives kept moving the victim from one district to another to avoid Swedi the sleuth, but he finally overtook them just after the sick man had died. Despite threats from the relatives, Swedi took blood smears from the body. Swedi was the person who discovered that the tsetse fly *G. swynnertoni* differed from *G. morsitans*. He was the one who observed that deciduous thicket served as a barrier to *morsitans*. For his work, the governor of Tanganyika awarded him the Certificate of Honour and Badge, the highest honor in Tanganyika to which Africans of those days could aspire.

As early as World War I, fly boys on instruction from their

chiefs were taking stationary positions in the bush, recording the number of flies they caught, and expressing these numbers in terms of flies per manhour. One of Swynnerton's entomologists, Dr. W. H. Potts, improved on this system in 1927; he conceived the idea of a fly round. To make a fly round Potts blazed a trail through the different types of vegetation he found in the area to be surveyed, then had three young Africans (fly boys) follow this trail. He divided the round into numbered sections, each of which corresponded to a vegetation type with the section number painted on a tree at the point of entry into that section. Walking through these vegetation types, the fly boys would stop every twenty yards to collect all the flies that settled either on themselves or on the ground around them. Sometimes they tabulated their catches as flies per worker-yard or, if the fly density was light, per worker per one hundred yards.

Potts's methods were widely adopted by other researchers. The first fly rounds, as the name would suggest, were circular courses so that fly boys could make full use of the return journey to headquarters, which a straight course out and back would not permit. To achieve greater accuracy in counts and wider knowledge of fly density and fly movements, the planners made fly rounds increasingly complex. Certain rounds were arranged to follow transect lines according to compass bearings. The greater accuracy that the transect lines afforded in establishing catching points and in judging fly populations compensated for the disadvantage of the unproductive return journey. Sometimes the fly round took on a rectilinear form; other times the rounds were organized as "octagonal spirals." In still other cases they became grids. One investigator designed a fly round covering almost four and one-half miles of pathways within a patch of ground no larger than a good-sized farm of approximately five hundred acres. Another researcher cut five fly rounds that totaled nearly thirty miles of pathways. The effort to assess accurately fly population within a given area got to the ridiculous point when too much fly rounding—too many fly boys traversing the area—actually changed the environment; it scared away host animals upon which the fly fed, the flies fled with the animals, and the excessive number of rounds defeated the purpose of obtaining accurate estimates of the original tsetse fly population density.

Later on, patrols of fly boys made rounds on bicycles. This proved to be another satisfactory method of taking a fly census since moving objects attracted flies. When feasible, teams making a fly density survey over an area resorted to car reconnaissance. A catching party on foot could go two miles an hour through country lightly infested with the fly; a truck could travel twelve to twenty miles per hour over roadless savanna country with two or three fly boys standing on the back of the truck catching flies as the vehicle moved along, calling out species, sex, and other characteristics of the tsetse they caught so that these data could be recorded and tabulated by the supervisor.

On some fly rounds done on foot, an ox was used as a bait animal to draw flies to the trail. This sort of lure was particularly useful where tsetse appeared to be little interested in man. In Zanzibar fly boys used bait oxen quite successfully to attract the species *G. austeni* to their fly round. They found this species of tsetse, which was thought to be rare, actually quite abundant over the area they were surveying.

Simple techniques on which the broad strategies of tsetse and trypanosome management depended sometimes turned into strategies themselves. Catching flies by hand, for instance, which developed to such a high degree of sophistication in the fly round as a method of assessing fly populations and movements, got put to good use to eradicate sleeping sickness. Obviously this technique could not be employed in a practical way over all of the four and one-half million square miles of Africa that the tsetse flies occupied. Indeed, the wonder was that catching flies by hand could be effective at all in preventing sleeping sickness. And yet the catch, or "swat-a-fly," procedure had its place in certain geographical areas where *G. palpalis,* the riverine species of tsetse, was restricted and precise in its habitat. Using this method, fly boys became key agents in destroying *G. palpalis* populations and in stamping out sleeping sickness from pockets where it was severe in Nigeria, in Kenya, and in the Sudan.

Along the Yuba River in southern Sudan, where the Zande people live, *G. palpalis,* which had invaded the area from the Congo, transmitted sleeping sickness to the people. In the early 1930's the government (Anglo-Egyptian condominium) succeeded in getting these people to move back from the river and leave the banks to the fly, and they urged the people to keep the land clear around their new villages so that they would remain free of flies. While these measures worked, they were not entirely satisfactory. Clearings grew back to bush, and the people drifted back to their former homesites along the river.

In 1938, when the incidence of sleeping sickness along the Yuba River was about sixty-five new cases per year and rising, the government started a scheme to bring the flies of the entire Yuba River and its tributaries under control with a three-year program using the hand-catching method. The supervisors of this project divided the river into six large blocks, each separated from the other by a clearing 800 yards long and 400 yards wide. The river coursed through the middle of the clearing, leaving 200 yards of cleared land on either side. The longer the clearing along the river, the harder for *G. palpalis* to move from one block to the next. The width mattered not so much, for *G. palpalis* rarely prospected for its hosts more than ten yards from the river's edge. Paths were cut on both sides of the river as close to the water as possible, up and down the tributaries as well as along the main stream. Each block was divided into sections; six to ten fly boys patrolled a section with a senior fly boy in charge. A group leader who had a fair knowledge of English and was up to the standard of a good hospital dresser of the medical profession of that day supervised all of the sections in a single block.

The fly boys, who in this case were eleven to sixteen years of age, lived in camps in the bush near their work. They started early in the morning with a period of physical exercises and worked until mid-afternoon. They received fifteen piastres (about fifty cents) a month plus clothing for their services. School grounds were provided for them, but from their earnings they built their own school buildings and paid for their books. At the height of the campaign 250 fly boys caught tsetse in the area. There was a long waiting list of those who wanted the job.

The flies each boy caught were tallied daily and added up at the end of the month. The fly boys who caught the most flies won money prizes. The competition was so keen that stealing one another's flies became a problem.

When the scheme started, the fly density along the Yuba River was so great that each fly boy caught about fifty flies a week. The program advanced, the number of flies each boy caught in a week dropped rapidly, and toward the close of the campaign in 1942 the number came to less than five. By 1942 new cases of sleeping sickness also dropped to approximately two per year, from the former sixty-five. When in 1940 it appeared that fly catching as a control measure on the Yuba River was working, the supervisors relaxed the regulations imposed on the people in the area. Those tribal groups dissatisfied with their new homes in the clearing along the roadway could and did move back in the bush by the river. Local clearings around villages were abandoned, and the people needed only to keep the main barriers cleared between blocks. The disease did not return.

Thousands of flies, tsetse flies, still die in Africa every day, at the hands of people who exercise no alternative but to slap them barehanded in desperation from their annoyance and bites. Thousands of flies meet the same end crushed by fly swatters. In one experiment alone, conducted from July 1946 to June 1947 in Kenya, a team of five African tsetse workers swatted 24,540 flies which they spotted on the trains they policed at the little towns of Emali and Sultan Hamud. These towns lay on the railroad route from Mombasa to Nairobi where the trains were going up-country from fly belt to fly-free territory. Involuntary reactions and emergency tactics such as those for fly survey and control worked under special conditions, but man had to exercise additional ingenuity if he were to control the fly on a grand scale.

In Zululand, part of the province of Natal in South Africa, a problem was arising because the farming population and particularly the cattle herders were pressing closer each year to the Umfolozi game reserve. The game in that sanctuary was also increasing in population and spreading by leaps and bounds; the animals ranged far beyond the borders of the reserve. Tsetse flies followed the game, intermingled with the cattle, and spread nagana to them. The Natal Provincial Administration had to take action.

An obscure entomologist, Dr. R. H. T. P. Harris, working for the Natal Provincial Administration (NPA) from 1920 to 1926, had argued that whatever control measures for tsetse were adopted it was necessary drastically to reduce the numbers of game animals as a preliminary step. Fly density was greatest in the game reserves where the largest number of game animals

were to be found. But by the time Harris had come to this con-
clusion he also realized that destroying game indiscriminately
would only cause the fly to hunt for its food more widely and to
extend its range into areas not yet infested. Thus the Natal government was persuaded to finance a scheme of organized shooting aimed at reducing the numbers of game animals to the
carrying capacity of the reserves and then to create a buffer
zone around the reserves completely free of both game and fly.

The buffer zone around the Umfolozi game reserve was divided into seven sections. A European ranger was assigned to
each; he had under his supervision "ten skilled native shots."
From May 1929 until November 1930 they destroyed 26,000
head of game in the buffer zone alone. These were, in the
words of Harris, "chiefly of zebra, wart-hog, duiker, and bush-
buck, all of which, by reason of their numbers and rapid increase, might have been placed in the category of vermin."

The slaughter in the buffer zone was necessary because the
tsetse population, like the game it attacked, comprised two
classes, a mobile and an immobile population. When game took
up a temporary abode in a new area, the tsetse that followed it
did likewise. The transient females of this population deposited
their larvae in the adopted areas. Their progeny became a new
immobile "garrison." Later the adults which emerged attacked
man, for the game had moved on. This was one way in which
tsetse extended its range. The growth and coalescence of such
garrisons formed fly belts. Classifying game populations the
same way, Harris believed that young game bred in buffer
zones must be killed. If not, these animals would return to their
birthplaces and establish an immobile population bringing new
flies with them to repopulate the zone freed of fly.

Keeping buffer zones free of game, however, became too expensive for the Natal Provincial Administration to continue.
They abandoned the project and allowed game and fly to move
back into the buffer zones adjacent to the farming areas.

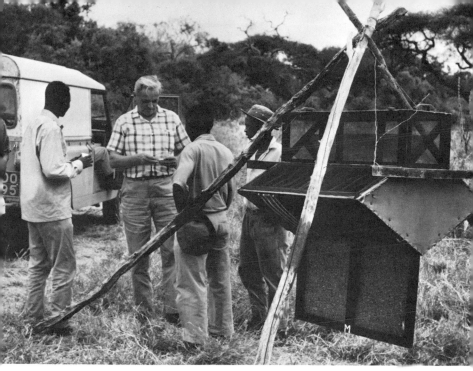

Examining the catch from a Harris fly trap; one side is open. (Photograph by Ordway Starnes.)

Besides the expense, the game destruction program suffered from other serious flaws. Absence of game stimulated hungry flies to disperse farther and wider than they ordinarily traveled. Harris had to look for ways to catch this population before it dispersed. Moreover, too many flies had to be caught for him to rely on fly boys to get the job done. And the inexorable temptation to replace manual work and individual care with gadgets was also operating.

Harris and others thought that a type of trap might work better than fly boys in attracting flies to be killed and in collecting data. He had noticed that tsetse depended on sight and on reactions to light values when in search of food. *G. pallidipes*, Bruce's fly, seemed well adapted to bush country because the changing light values in the bush stimulated it to travel and to hunt. Later workers believed that Harris oversimplified in emphasizing the fly's reaction to light. Nevertheless the trap he built based on his observations serves today with but slight modifications to collect this fly in astronomical numbers from the game reserves and wherever else it is abundant.

The Harris trap, if one stretched his imagination, resembled the body of an animal. Field men hung the trap low under a tree, where it benefited from light shade and constant motion which attracted tsetse. A wooden platform six feet long served as the back. Two frames covered with burlap hanging down and sloping inward made up the sides. From the end, the body looked like an inverted triangle. The underside, which might resemble an animal's belly, was left open with a six-inch gap its full length to admit flies searching for a vulnerable place to feed. The top or the back of the trap supported a wire cage on top which ran its full length. Flies moving down to the underside of the trap would enter the slit, move up inside the body and then through another narrow slit into the screen cage. When attacking an animal, tsetse flies will drive or dart to its belly and then dart back into the sunlight. They will do the same when approaching the trap. Once in the trap they are drawn to the light at the top and are not likely to escape through the dark slit below.

The trap was a great success. The Natal Provincial Administration ordered a thousand traps for the Umfolozi game reserve. The traps caught flies in such numbers in the summer of 1931 that they had to be counted by the quart jar. Nine hundred and eighty-three traps were set by September 1931, and during that month the traps at peak load captured 2,088,508 flies. From September the fly population declined sharply and it looked as though here was one situation where a whole campaign might be based simply on the use of traps.

But financial stringency in January 1932 broke the incipient campaign, all work stopped, and for three months the thousand traps, all finally erected, went unattended. Ants and spiders got into the cages. Heavy rains fell causing a rank growth of vegetation around the traps, screening them from flies. In April the NPA staff was restored to fifty per cent of its previous strength but it could no longer assess with accuracy the value of the abandoned traps.

Some idea of trap efficacy came, however, from Harris, who wrote that during the summer months of 1931 flies had been so numerous in the Umfolozi reserve that one had to close all the windows of his car when he drove through in order to keep from being bitten severely. One trap there that June captured nearly seven thousand flies. A year later the total fly catch of the same trap at this same place did not exceed ninety, and some traps in the area caught no flies at all. Later workers discovered that the Harris trap was extremely effective when the tsetse was abundant but not so useful when the fly population was low. Probably it never would have served as the sole agent for the control and possible eradication of tsetse. Moreover, while the Harris trap worked well for this one species of tsetse, *G. pallidipes,* it did very little to capture *G. morsitans* or *G. palpalis,* the most important sleeping sickness carrier.

Harris's pioneer work encouraged others to build traps, too. Swynnerton devised a screen for trapping flies, and one of the workers in his program invented a round cylinder which when covered with crinoline was supposed to convince tsetse it might be the size and shape of a man. Electric traps, traps with fans, and a host of other types met with variable success on the game and savanna species of fly, but *G. palpalis* and its companion *G. tachinoides,* so important in West Africa for the spread of sleeping sickness, remained elusive.

In 1930 a man-and-wife team, Dr. K. R. S. Morris and his wife Marjory, invented a trap that proved to be reliable for both these species. Tsetse depended mainly upon goats as a reservoir of food in northern Ghana, so the Morrises fashioned their trap to resemble a goat. Further, their trap had to lure tsetse in the sacred groves along the riverbanks of the intermittent streams where animals and man communed. The sacred groves were "national parks," the "green belts" for the nearby congested villages. Rigorous taboos opposed cutting any vegetation in them, so that to practice clearing techniques would have been very unpopular. One or two attempts to clear such groves had already cost the confidence and cooperation of the people. Morris had hired fly boys who, in hand-catching flies, had rapidly reduced the tsetse fly population in these groves in a matter of eight to ten weeks. But the odd fly or two left or introduced again in a grove would always remain a potential nucleus of a new population. Morris tried Harris, Swynnerton, and many other traps, but they did not work, so he built ones of his own design. He, too, found that the essential features of a trap were the highlights and shadows that played over its upper and lower surfaces. He built his trap to look like the torso of an animal and to be conspicuous when viewed from any angle. His work, in effect, was an exercise in building a scarecrow to attract rather than to frighten its quarry. At first Morris used animal skins complete with head, tail, and legs, to make the trap rather like a miniature Trojan horse. But soon he discovered that the entomologist more than the tsetse appreciated this degree of naturalism. When he simplified his trap, it looked like a drum or brown cylinder with four legs below and a cage on top, the cylinder covered with skin, the legs sunk into the ground so that the bulk of the trap would only be about a foot above the ground, the same in height as a goat, in order to catch the maximum number of tsetse. His traps did not have to be hung from trees and in constant motion from winds, as those set for *G. pallidipes* in South African game country had to be. *G. palpalis* and *G. tachinoides* in West Africa preferred a stationary trap.

Fly boys (trap boys) would carry them by bicycle, sometimes three at a time, find an appropriate site, and set them up. On their rounds they would bring along hammer and nails, needle and thread, and spare cloth to make minor repairs if necessary. Snakes or lizards might enter the traps at times, but these were usually harmless. Damage was infrequent. Vandalism seldom occurred, although occasionally little boys who liked to use the traps as targets for their arrows would slash or puncture them. No doubt Morris felt that he had really arrived when one of his traps so simulated the small game and goats of the region that an enthusiastic hunter successfully stalked and shot one covered by a duiker skin.

Some flies, after wandering over the body of the Morris trap, made their way upward and flew away instead of working their way down under the belly and moving up through the opening to its insides. An awning put over the top to project outward and slightly downward in order to capture such flies did not help because the awning spoiled the effect of contrasting light and shadow. It also obscured visibility of the trap from a distance. Morris built large traps, too, but the flies really preferred goat-size ones except for those double in size, raised to about shoulder height, and patterned roughly after the size of the local dwarf cattle. Such traps attracted a fair number of tsetse. Eventually goat, sheep, and small antelope skins, which were scarce, relatively expensive, and subject to rot during the rainy season, were replaced by black cloth, khaki drill, or burlap. Materials of rough texture attracted more flies than smooth ones, and open feeding grounds were better as sites for traps than thickets where the fly bred. They did well in areas where man was a principal host, along riverbanks, at ferries, bridges and fords, water holes, washing places, or animal drinking places. The regular presence of hosts in considerable numbers led to prolific trapping, and a trap placed close to the real hosts would yield the highest catches. But traps so placed were liable to be upset or pushed aside. Traps placed at right angles to the general flow of flies along the river banks would intercept more hungry flies on their way to feed than traps pointed along the line of flight.

Whatever their size, shape, color, and placement, traps set out in great numbers required a lot of hand labor, which fly boys performed successfully. But it still remained necessary, as it had always been, to probe for new ways to combat this pest; poisoning flies looked exceedingly promising.

One might have thought that the African people would have developed diabolical insect poisons long, long ago; they concocted amazingly effective poisons to apply to arrow tips directed against wild game and their enemies. Yet hardly anywhere in the world, let alone in Africa, did people develop insect poisons until the nineteenth century, when they began to use stomach poisons like lead arsenate and contact ones like nicotine and pyrethrum; during that century they surged into prominence. These chemicals are called "first-generation" pesticides in modern parlance.

DDT, short for dichloro-diphenyl-trichloro-ethane, and its chlorinated hydrocarbon relatives appeared on the scene about the time of World War II as phenomenally effective pesticides, when insects were building up resistance to the first-generation pesticides. These chemicals, "second-generation" pesticides in Harvard Professor Carroll Williams' terminology, made the poison technique of killing flies a nearly universal practice. At the close of World War II the abundant availability of surplus DDT enabled experimenters to apply that insecticide to a wide variety of insect pests; tsetse flies were no exception.

To apply a dash of poison, a residual one which remains active for months on everything the fly is likely to touch, puts time and space between the exterminator and the victim. This technique enables one to avoid facing his enemy and making a messy kill; he can sprinkle poison over tsetse breeding grounds and resting sites, leave these, and wait at a distance for the fly to contact the poison and for the poison to take effect. This is easy for those who are squeamish. It waters down the responsibility for the actual kill and salves one's conscience, if indeed he worries about killing a fly.

Two philosophies conflicted over how to direct a squirt of spray or a poof of dust against tsetse. One advocated broadcasting the poison widely and indiscriminately; the other, putting it selectively where it would do the most good.

During the late 1940's some experimenters directed DDT to the source of food and thus rather specifically at adult flies. In Swynnerton territory, they used old Shinyanga block four, parts A and B, which covered five square miles of thorn bush, where G. pallidipes dominated, although G. swynnertoni also occupied the area. Bait cattle which were sprayed with poison were deployed in the bush at a ratio of six oxen to one member of the larger game species in order to exhaust the fly population as rapidly as possible. Oxen were used because among domesticated stock they were the favored hosts of the fly. Suggestive of subsequent experiments to reduce fly populations by liberating sterile male flies to compete with fertile ones over an area, the whole idea depended upon the supposedly greater attractiveness of cattle than of game to the flies. The oxen were dosed with drugs—phenidium, for example—to protect them from trypanosomiasis, and thus they could be kept in the bush for considerable lengths of time. If the oxen were sprayed with a solution of 9-per-cent pure DDT and resin in groundnut oil once a week, 70 per cent of the flies which alighted on them died; sprayed twice a week, 95 per cent of the flies succumbed.

Herded in batches of tens over a ten-hour day for a ten-month period of time, the oxen as walking bags of poison reduced the female tsetse population 70 per cent over the whole area. Five years later in an area close by a similar experiment, refined, gave better results than the one carried out in block four.

But the objective, fly extermination, was never achieved, for both experiments underestimated the vitality of the fly. In the second experiment, the irreducible minimum population that remained was capable of explosive growth. New flies from adjacent places migrated to the experimental area. In the earlier experiment *G. pallidipes* fed at night when the oxen were not around; the heavy thorn bush obstructed the cattle's visibility. Often the fly did not find the cattle: only 13 per cent to 25 per cent of the flies actually came to the oxen. Nevertheless, the poison bait system allowed for an economy of materials over a wide area and it lessened the widespread and incalculable effect of insecticide application on the general wild plant and animal community.

When judiciously used, DDT, dieldrin, and similar chemicals maligned today for their noxious overall effect gave spectacular results in poisoning flies with very little apparent harm to the total environment. In 1960 the Veterinary Tsetse and Trypanosomiasis Unit of what was then the Northern Region of Nigeria carried out a partial spraying program along the Kibori River not far from the site of Nash's Anchau scheme. This minor tributary of the Kaduna River was small and narrow with an understory of shrubs and creepers extending back only fifteen feet from the river bank. The total length of the Kibori River was just sixteen miles, including its subsidiary branches. The shrubs and creepers constituted a dense wall of vegetation breached only at water crossings, at cattle watering points, and at places where man had cleared land for small banana and ginger farms. Farther back from the banks, repeated clearing

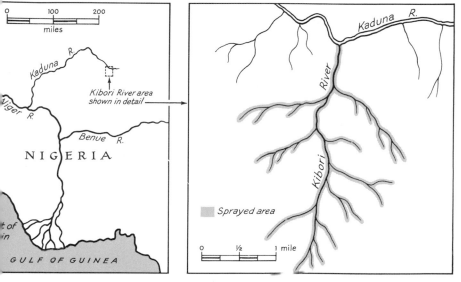

Spot-map of the Kibori River, Nigeria. (Drawn by John Morris.)

turned the normal woodlands into scrublands. Intensified shifting cultivation transformed some of the scrubland into permanent blocks of farmland.

G. palpalis hovered in large numbers in the shady humid groves close to the village water holes and at other places where men and their cattle crossed the river. If these areas were sprayed during February, March, and late in the dry season, the entire tsetse population would come into contact with the insecticide left on the vegetation, for the flies alit on it to wait there to feed upon cattle or, having already fed, to excrete body fluids immediately after the blood meal.

A pair of laborers, each with a knapsack mist-blower strapped to his back, sprayed the vegetation with a 2-per-cent dieldrin mixture made by adding one part of a 20-per-cent dieldrin concentrate to nine parts of river water. An auxiliary team of insecticide carriers and insecticide mixers followed the spray team. A fully trained tsetse control assistant supervised the operations at all times.

The spraymen walked along the outer margins of the vegetation on each riverbank. When they came to a gap, a concentration site for flies, they went down to the riverbed and sprayed the lower four feet of all of the shade-forming vegetation immediately adjacent to and bordering it. Then they returned to the margins of the vegetation and continued along the banks until they came to another break in the marginal vegetation bordering the river.

Within twenty-four hours after spraying, the entire tsetse population collapsed; it never recovered. Tsetse control officers knew this because they had deployed patrols to count flies. At the beginning of the experiment the patrols collected an average of ten flies per visit at the collection sites. Ten months after the treatments the patrols could not find a single fly in the places sprayed.

The Kibori River eradication program exemplifies a judicious use of a deadly weapon not to destroy but to enhance the quality of the environment. It obviated the need to continue with a slash-burn program, or even to undertake discriminative clearing of riverbank vegetation. One of those persistent pesticides now banned for use in certain parts of the world proved to be less disruptive to the environment than the traditional techniques. Selective and cheap, it drew for its efficacy upon sound knowledge of the pest in relation to its environment.

Dieldrin came to the rescue of a faltering fly-eradication program in the old Ankole region of southwestern Uganda. *G. morsitans,* the game fly, had expanded northward and crossed the Kagera River—the border between Karagwe and Ankole

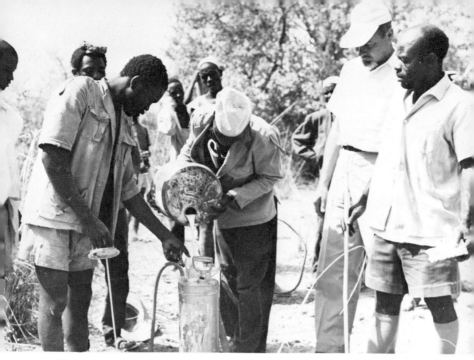

Filling a knapsack sprayer for use in a tsetse control campaign in northern Nigeria. (Photograph from United States Agency for International Development, 1964.)

—at the turn of the century. Rinderpest, one will recall, had invaded the area and decimated the cattle population, leaving the starving tsetse fly population no alternative but to contract toward the river. By the late 1920's the population of flies recovered, expanded north, and again reached the Mbarara-Masaka road, the main east-west highway across the country. Clearing strips of land as barriers to prevent tsetse from advancing failed. By 1951 tsetse occupied 260 square miles north of the road. Instituted in 1952, discriminative clearing of bush also lacked full effectiveness, although it had reduced the infestation. By 1957 tsetse had advanced another 750 square miles; discriminative clearing was abandoned. The fly spread rapidly toward Toro to the north and Buganda to the east. In July 1958 the Uganda Tsetse Control Department decided upon a game-shooting campaign to reduce the food supply of tsetse, to do with a gun what rinderpest as a virus did at the turn of the century. All but 5,000 of the 65,000 cattle in the area were moved out to reduce further tsetse's food supply. These drastic measures notwithstanding, the fly not only survived, it spread and succeeded in crossing the Katonga River into Toro. Toward the end of 1959 in desperation, the Uganda Tsetse Control Department resorted to spraying a solution of poison along a barrier zone a half-mile wide on the Toro side of the Katonga River; this halted the advance. Game hunting within the area continued to reduce the fly population, but it evoked protest from conservationists and others.

To eliminate the fly from the last six hundred square miles of the area, in 1962 the Tsetse Control Department, by then called the Uganda Tsetse Control Division, decided to turn to insecticides again. Dr. W. R. Wooff had become Chief Tsetse Officer, and he reported directly to the vice president of Uganda. The facts, figures, and capacity at his command enabled him to draw from the Uganda government adequate funds, equipment, and manpower to get on with a successful job of eradicating tsetse. His operations required a budget of $1.5 million per year. He commanded his men as though he were general of an army; each wore a uniform. Four Ugandans who were senior civil servants worked under his direction; they and other subordinate staff were devoted to him.

To eradicate tsetse from the six hundred square miles of Ankole, Dr. Wooff had to organize a "tracks and camp unit" for constructing many miles of roadways in order to make the entire area accessible by motor vehicles and to divide it into manageable blocks. Then he assembled knapsack sprayer squads to enter the blocks and to apply poison to the resting sites of the savanna species of fly, *G. morsitans,* from ground level up into the branches of the thorn trees to a height of ten feet. The spray teams used sprayers with special extension lances and nozzles in order properly to place the 3-per-cent dieldrin emulsion they used on vegetation.

The tsetse operations might impress one as being, after all, quite routine. Not so. In the early 1960's, as in years past, such operations offered their fair share of excitement, much of it depending upon personalities. An English entomologist of great ability, Dr. Wooff let his personality expand beyond the stereotype impression one is likely to hold of scientists always objective in their thought and action. Dr. Wooff is slightly built, blue-eyed; he wears gold-rimmed spectacles. When he shakes your hand, he bows and curtly clicks his heels. Ask him why he came to Uganda to engage in tsetse control—his answer: to hunt elephants. But this disarming reply does not hint at his sound knowledge of tsetse and his qualities of leadership. His administration was a lively one.

Since 1962, when Uganda gained its independence, power struggles had been going on between the tribes of the north and the Baganda people who cultivate their plantain and coffee around the borders of Lake Victoria. The Baganda, traditionally the aristocrats, lost ground in the struggle; their ruler, the Kabaka, who was descended from King Mtesa, whom Stanley, Lord Lugard, and other explorers knew, was exiled. This created tension amounting to a national emergency. Curfews were imposed on the nation, and travel from one part of the country to another became dangerous. Dr. Wooff, traveling for the government on an official tour of duty, met a roadblock set by the Baganda people to halt any vehicle or person of government or official character. Wooff's mission was urgent and important. When he attempted to press on, tempers became frazzled. Right or wrong, goaded into action or not, Wooff drew his pistol, shot into the crowd and infuriated them. Many were armed with pangas; they slashed up Wooff and his assistant and left them for dead. But Wooff and his companion recovered after a stretch in the hospital. They continued with dedication and drive to command the tsetse eradication operations of the Uganda government. Significantly, the Uganda government placed highest priority on the talent and the dedication that the director of the tsetse fly control unit displayed in this instance and thereby extended a tolerance for irrational actions that might not have been obtained to the same extent under other circumstances.

The postwar period, in which directing a dash of poison to flies in specific localities was a popular method of insect control, also witnessed broadcasting by air great quantities of poison over vast areas of Africa. Many a World War II pilot suddenly found himself mustered out of the air force with nothing to do and became a bush pilot. Bush pilots, surplus planes, and vast quantities of surplus DDT made it possible for men to find out what insecticides really would do when blanketed over fly belts. Islands in Lake Victoria, valleys of Rwanda, plains of Tanzania, and game reserves of South Africa became prime targets for grand-scale experiments, which were sometimes designed with reckless disregard for the environment, to put tsetse to bed for good.

The first of the airplane application experiments took place in Zululand in South Africa in 1947 following an exceptionally severe outbreak of nagana; it took seven years to complete. The objective was to eradicate the fly, especially *G. pallidipes,* at whatever cost. Airplane dusting or spraying constituted simply one more tool added to those already in use: game destruction, bush clearing, firing the land, and trapping adult flies.

Special conditions prevailed over this area of seven thousand square miles. *G. pallidipes* was already isolated in an ecological pocket; it had no contact with its relatives of the same species in the north. In Zululand it bred in some areas and foraged in others. Once this was understood, it followed that if an extermination campaign killed all the flies at the breeding sites, there could be no foraging flies. The breeding sites, coincident with the game reserves, embraced but 3 per cent of the total area.

The South Africans called DDT into service first. Later they relied on the cheaper and equally effective poison lindane, which is another of the chlorinated hydrocarbons. They diluted technical grade DDT with ordinary furnace oil to get a 5-per-cent final concentration. Pilots flew six surplus military aircraft at a time over the experimental area in echelon formation and at a height of only fifty to seventy-five feet above the ground. They literally strafed tsetse with the 5-per-cent DDT. Each plane delivered atomized insecticide in a swath approximately 210 feet wide, but the atomized insecticide was practically invisible and the pilots had great difficulty telling which strips of countryside they had sprayed and which remained for them to cover. They solved this problem when they introduced the insecticide in liquid form directly into the engine exhaust, where the blast of hot exhaust gases vaporized the liquid to the extent that it emerged as a dense white smoke.

At the peak of the operations, Piper Cruiser airplanes replaced the heavier military aircraft. These single-engined planes, lined up eight abreast, spewed BHC over 30,000 acres of land per month. Each plane could travel over fifteen acres per minute, but only at the dawn of four mornings a week on the average could pilots expect the windless conditions essential to lay the smoke carefully and effectively on the land. Over rough terrain, pilots flew helicopters as close to the treetops as was possible, but in some really heavily bushed valleys the topography made it too hazardous to fly and too difficult to gain good penetration of the vegetation from the air. Here men or boys, called "generator boys," traveling on foot placed at seventy-yard intervals hand grenades which when ignited generated atomized insecticide to kill the flies.

In Zululand the aerial application of insecticides seems to have achieved the practical eradication of tsetse. Such clear-cut results do not come out of experiments with airplane application of insecticides in other areas, and though there appear to be no adverse ecological effects, this question needs to be studied. In Tanzania, problems cropped up in laying the insecticide properly over the landscape in order to get it in contact with the tsetse. In other areas, the high cost of aerial application made the method prohibitive. So "kill the fly" efforts must continue with a smorgasbord choice to be made among all of the standard techniques ranging from the fly swatter to airplane application of poison. New methods must continually be devised.

Refinements on the use of a dash of poison now go well beyond a squirt of spray or a poof of dust to the habitat of the fly. In an experimental way, David A. Dame and his associates from the United States tried to eradicate tsetse from an area in Rhodesia by sterilizing male flies with a chemical called tepa. Sterilized male flies when liberated would mate with the females in nature; they would compete with the fertile male population not so treated. If present in large enough numbers, sterile males would send the fly population on a downward curve to extinction.

In the mid-1960's scientists discovered a growth-preventing pesticide in paper. Now one can imagine such headlines for tsetse as "eat the daily newspaper and die." Carroll M. Williams of Harvard and Karel Slama from Prague found that this growth-preventing substance is a constituent of newsprint. It resembles the "juvenile hormone" of insects which "staves off metamorphosis" and obstructs the transformation of larvae to adults. This constituent has been traced through paper pulp to balsam trees. Ferns may have it too. Entomologists call this substance an ecdysone because it regulates when and if an insect will molt, that is, go through ecdysis. It qualifies as a "third-generation" or biological pesticide, a selective one perhaps to replace a pesticide like DDT, which is nonselective.

But entomologists cannot stop. They must continually explore new possibilities; their arsenal of chemicals must be well-nigh inexhaustible. They may ultimately isolate and synthesize the sex attractants of flies that govern reproduction, manufacture them and liberate them in sufficient quantities to confuse the flies and upset their mating procedures. Or, as the American entomologists E. F. Knipling and Carroll M. Williams point out, they may use such substances to attract male flies, which then can be treated with a chemosterilant; when the flies are released, they can transmit this sterilant venereally to their mates and again shatter the potential of the fly to increase in numbers.

In David Livingstone's time, the approach to combating communicable diseases was similar to that of the witch's cooking up a charm in Shakespeare's *Macbeth:*

> *1 Witch.* Round about the cauldron go;
> In the poison'd entrails throw. . . .
> *2 Witch.* Fillet of a fenny snake,
> In the cauldron boil and bake;
> Eye of newt, and toe of frog,
> Wool of bat, and tongue of dog;
> Adder's fork, and blind-worm's sting,
> Lizard's leg, and howlet's wing;
> For a charm of pow'rful trouble,
> Like a hell-broth boil and bubble. . . .
> *All.* Double, double, toil and trouble;
> Fire burn, and cauldron bubble.

2 Witch. Cool it with a baboon's blood;
Then the charm is firm and good.

A physician could do little better than the son of a Batoka chief who, more than a century ago, gave Livingstone and his brother a recipe to cure tsetse-bitten cattle. He told them to take the bark of a certain root and a dozen tsetse flies dried and ground together in a fine powder, to administer some of the mixture internally, and then to fumigate the cattle by burning the rest of it under them. He suggested that they continue the treatment for weeks whenever the symptoms of nagana appeared. He freely admitted that the recipe would not cure every sick beast, but he thought that in most cases it helped and hoped that if the Livingstones thought so, too, perhaps in their travels they would send presents back to him in return for his disclosure. For a strange echo of this recipe in our time see the accompanying comic strip.

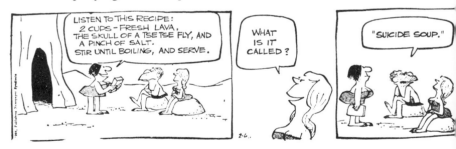

Suicide soup, "B.C." cartoon. (By permission of John Hart and Field Enterprises, Inc.)

Chieftain, cartoonist, or chemist—someone had to concoct a recipe for a soup that trypanosomes could "quaff" with suicidal results but which would be innocuous to man and beast. Starting out hit-or-miss, chemists and pharmacologists gradually narrowed the search for effective drugs and devised systematic ways to look for new ones. As we have seen, the star ingredient in this process was arsenic.

The trouble with arsenic, as the deaths and blindness it caused in the early years showed, was that it was devastating and nondiscriminating. It attacked host and parasite with equal vigor. Chemists had to bind arsenic to some organic compound that would not let it ionize—that is, float freely in the host and combine with elements there that would result in damage to the host. The vehicle chemical itself had to have rigid specifications that would enable it to distribute the arsenic through blood and tissue, to deliver it safely to the disease agents, and then free it to penetrate and destroy them.

In a sense, the taming of arsenic really started in the search for a way to synthesize quinine. A brilliant young chemist, William Perkin, working in England in 1856 tried to make the antimalarial drug from aniline but got a beautiful mauve-color substance instead. Realizing the potential of his discovery as a dye, he abandoned any further efforts to synthesize quinine and devoted his attention to the aniline dye industry, which developed from his discovery. The rapid growth of this industry set a French chemist, Pierre Jacques Antoine Béchamp, to work trying to make an oxidant to produce the brilliant bluish-red dye fuchsin. He heated arsenic with aniline in 1863 and got a compound, subsequently called atoxyl, which he thought to be a salt, aniline arsenate.

A leading German chemist, Paul Ehrlich, who had made notable contributions to dye chemistry and immunology, tested atoxyl's action against trypanosomes around the turn of the century. As a trypanocide, atoxyl had lain on the shelf for a number of years after Béchamp had synthesized it, just as DDT was discovered in 1876 but not recognized for its insecticidal properties until the 1940's. Before 1900, who even knew a trypanocide was needed? Unfortunately the strain of parasite

Ehrlich was using happened to be arsenic resistant, so he got negative results.

But in 1905 H. Wolferstan Thomas and Anton Breinl in Liverpool found atoxyl to be effective against another strain of trypanosomes in dosages that were nonlethal to host animals. The report surprised Ehrlich because it contradicted what he would have expected on the basis of atoxyl's reported chemical structure. Béchamp had thought that if atoxyl were a salt, it would readily break down into ions in a man's body. In this form, with nothing to attach the arsenic specifically to the parasite, the poison would be expected to damage the host as much as the microorganism. Ehrlich rushed to Liverpool, confirmed the results of Thomas and Breinl, returned to Germany, and with his colleague Alfred Bertheim reanalyzed atoxyl. The formula Béchamp had proposed was wrong. Atoxyl was not aniline arsenate but rather the sodium salt of arsanilic acid and held arsenic tightly in its molecule so that it would not readily come apart in the bloodstream. Ehrlich's investigation of atoxyl's action led to the development of many other trypanocidal compounds and, in fact, established him as the father of the science of chemotherapy, the treatment of communicable diseases with poisons that act against the infecting agent but not the host.

Following Robert Koch's work in East Africa atoxyl became the standard treatment for sleeping sickness. But it fell far short of being an ideal trypanocide. Rarely did it give a permanent cure; relapses of disease frequently occurred following its use. Painful to the patient after injection, it damaged the optic nerve if too much was administered. It had a narrow therapeutic index, that is, a small difference between the "curative" dose that would kill trypanosomes in human blood and the "tolerated" dose beyond which the host would suffer damage. And when left in the light for some time it decomposed, becoming even more toxic to human beings.

After examining 605 other arsenical compounds, Ehrlich went on to synthesize salvarsan arsphenamine. Though when mishandled it sometimes caused death, salvarsan became a powerful control for syphilis. It did nothing chemically for sleeping sickness, but indirectly the excitement over its discovery had great impact. When World War I threatened to interrupt the flow to the United States of synthetic dyes and of salvarsan from Germany, the prime producer, Americans feared that there might be no more salvarsan to combat syphilis. Two chemists at the Rockefeller Institute for Medical Research, W. A. Jacobs and Michael Heidelberger, encouraged by their director Simon Flexner, set out to duplicate Ehrlich's salvarsan (which they did) *and concurrently to look for trypanocides more effective than atoxyl.* The quest for effective but safe chemicals for the control of African sleeping sickness had reached the United States. From 1914 until 1919, Heidelberger and Jacobs screened innumerable arsenicals specifically to find a substitute for atoxyl. They chose to alter atoxyl rather than salvarsan because of the "bondage" properties of arsenic. Chemically, arsenic has its bonds of strength, called valence, which govern the number of atoms or groups of atoms that will cling to it; these are set by natural law at either three or five. The five-bonded, or pentavalent, arsenic in atoxyl happened to be more stable, more water-soluble, and more diffusible than the trivalent arsenic in salvarsan, though the trivalent form can be much more effective once it reaches the scene of action.

In 1917, Jacobs and Heidelberger synthesized tryparsamide, short for TRYPanosome-ARSenic-AMIDE. They had taken one of Ehrlich's arsenicals, replaced its carboxyl (-COOH) group with an amide, -$CONH_2$, which reduced its toxicity to host tissue. Rockefeller Institute pathologists Wade Hampton Brown and Louise Pearce obtained promising curative results in rabbits and mice infected with *Trypanosoma gambiense* and *T. brucei* in New York. Pearce then tried out tryparsamide in Leopoldville, the Belgian Congo, on seventy-seven patients suffering in the advanced stages of the Gambian form of the disease; it proved to be a tremendous improvement over atoxyl. For the first time a drug appeared to have a beneficial effect on late-stage sleeping sickness. More than 50 per cent of the patients with second-stage sleeping sickness improved through treatment with tryparsamide. But this drug, later widely used, like its predecessors constituted a threat to the optic nerve, as Albert Schweitzer and Eugène Jamot discovered. Moreover, strains of trypanosomes developed resistance to it.

In synthesizing tryparsamide the chemists still had not finished with arsenic. Over the next decade, 1922–1932, in many parts of the world they brought to approximately 12,500 the total number of arsenical compounds put together in order to arrive at just the right form in which to present this poison to the parasite and, at the same time, to make it less damaging than atoxyl or tryparsamide to the optic nerve.

Dr. Ernst A. H. Friedheim was one of these chemists. A Swiss who had worked in many parts of the world, he maintained private laboratories in New York in the 1930's. There he decided to associate sulfonic acid with atoxyl. He wanted to create a highly acid condition in the host tissue so that when the molecule did disassociate in the tissue the arsenic ion would not be likely to join up with the lipids of the brain and optic nerve, which preferred to combine with arsenic in an alkaline environment. Higher dosages of arsenic would then be possible before damage to the brain and the optic nerve would occur. This reasoning proved to be correct, and Friedheim produced some effective trypanocides this way. But treatment with them still required several weeks, and in search of a speedier drug Friedheim took another approach. Having noticed that all good trypanocides contained nitrogen in one form or another, he thought melamine chemistry might offer a convenient starting point for a trypanocide. In this chemistry, important in the manufacture of plastics, large numbers of nitrogen atoms would join to one of arsenic. It was melamine and arsenic that, joined together, gave him melarsen, which has six nitrogen atoms in its formula.

When Friedheim tried out melarsen in West Africa in 1938 it seemed effective. He discovered that, curiously, the tribal people along the coasts of West Africa tolerated dosages higher than those which an inland people, the Mossi, could stand. At first he reasoned that coastal people, being fisherman, had a much higher proportion of protein in their diet than did those sorghum, millet, and cassava eaters of sub-Saharan Africa, the Mossi. Therefore he suggested that the Mossi under melarsen treatment for *gambiense* sleeping sickness be fed large quantities of Swiss cheese. He found that this group of people could then tolerate dosages equivalent to the ones the fisherman could take. Quick to profit from these preliminary leads and from his earlier experience with sulfonic acid, Friedheim wondered whether the sulfur in the cheese, rather than the protein as such, made the difference. It did.

Next Friedheim tackled the potent trivalent arsenoxides from which Jacobs and Heidelberger had shied away. After several years of fruitless work he combined melarsen oxide and British Antilewisite, or BAL, a sulfur-bearing compound which had been developed as an antidote for the arsenical war gas lewisite during the war. This produced what he called Mel B, a great advance over melarsen. He went on to synthesize Mel W, which, being water soluble, was relatively easy to inject into the bloodstream.

Arsenic, for so many years a dangerous though effective try-panosome killer, had now become an orderly, selective poison. Hundreds of thousands of sleeping sickness victims owed their lives to this element when administered to them through Mel B, Mel W, and through their predecessor compounds. Throughout the long search for an appropriate arsenical, the helter-skelter procedure reminiscent of "Double, double, toil and trouble" underlay the "I told you so" logic of hindsight, imparting an apparently streamlined quality to the steps taken to make out of arsenic a therapeutic compound.

But ideas seemed exhausted for contriving other combinations of chemical substances that would bring arsenic to the pinnacle of perfection as a therapeutic agent. Even the newest arsenicals had their limitations. Mel B was curative only, not prophylactic; Mel W was somewhat toxic to patients. Sometimes the patients suffered relapses of the disease. Trypanosomes often developed tolerance to arsenic, and worst of all it never did effectively control the most virulent sleeping sickness agent, *T. rhodesiense*. For that reason arsenic became a tool for the differentiation of the two trypanosome species attacking man, *T. rhodesiense* and *T. gambiense*.

A number of chemists ignored arsenic at the height of its fame. They followed lines of research suggested by another development in Paul Ehrlich's laboratories, the dyes trypan red and trypan blue. Before working on atoxyl Ehrlich had found that trypan red killed some types of trypanosomes with a high therapeutic index, but it did not work against the species causing human and animal trypanosomiasis in Africa. Trypan blue did cure nagana in cattle, but it also dyed their tissues. When ultimately the cattle were slaughtered, who wanted to eat blue meat? Here the motivation, a dual one, was to find alternative compounds which would not turn meat blue and, of course, ones which would *effectively* kill trypanosomes. Bayer 205, a "colorless" dye also known as suramin and germanin, emerged from such studies. This compound, its formula long kept secret, acted like a dye in the way it congregated and precipitated around the trypanosomes. It also associated itself with blood proteins and did not, therefore, become easily eliminated by the kidneys. Since it blocked trypanosome activity and since it stayed in host tissue for some time, it had protective as well as curative value within its animal or human host.

In other ways, chemists searched beyond arsenic for materials that would make the best trypanocide. Friedheim replaced the arsenic in melarsen with the metallic element antimony and got a compound called MSb, which occurred in two forms. One form, small and distinctive, was a monomer—a single free molecule; the other was a polymer—its molecules strung together like a series of paper dolls. The former, being small like melarsen, was immediately toxic to the trypanosomes, but was rapidly eliminated through the host; it worked well as a cure but did not stay long enough in the body to be a preventative. The latter, being large and complicated when injected into muscle tissue, was sparingly soluble. It slowly broke down into monomers over a period of many months; it stayed in the host and therefore protected it over a period of time.

The antibiotics of the 1950's and 1960's were tested and screened for their efficacy against trypanosomes; none has as yet appeared particularly effective.

The decades of investigations that grew out of Ehrlich's work in immunology led to an understanding of immune reactions, of the antigens and the antibodies which govern the relationship of parasite to host. The vital question, why will not the body produce its own protective chemicals in sufficient amount to combat trypanosomes, still needed an answer. At long last, the answer may be on the horizon. The body produces the antibodies, but unfortunately trypanosomes seem quite capable of adjusting almost weekly to the challenge of these antibodies and to other modified host conditions; they turn up new strains of their own which thrive in the body, blood, and tissue. Nevertheless, recent studies as far distant from Africa as Washington, D.C., and confirmed in Glasgow, Scotland, brighten the outlook for creating a live vaccine that will protect cattle, if not yet human beings, from trypanosomiasis. Bombarding trypanosomes with radioactive cobalt alters them so that when injected into a suitable host they do not cause the disease but may still force the host to manufacture its own poisons to protect it from the onslaught of wild, natural strains of the disease organism—to concoct a murderous soup for the trypanosome.

V

"You Tell Me to Sit Quiet"

*The aim pursued is not to carry on research in splendid institutes
but to do more urgent work—to prevent men dying!*

P. Richet
*Control and Surveillance Techniques
in Human Trypanosomiasis*

As the fight against tsetse fly diseases changed from a desperate battle to check a rampant killer to a slow, long-range campaign, the framework of action became institutionalized. The campaign, depending on the time, place, situation, and colonial power involved, was entrusted to special commissions, both temporary and permanent, to action programs that engaged men in field operations, and to "splendid institutes" that drew men, money, and materials from European governments, singly and in cooperation, as well as from the colonies. Paralleling the institutionalization of science as a whole, research and technology on a fragile fly and its silent trypanosomes developed into a field in which men could reasonably expect to spend entire careers. These groups coalesced into a network, and the network, in the broadest sense, into an empire. In size, effort, and monies expended, this empire could not be matched in Africa by the parallel empires constructed around malaria, yellow fever, and their whispering mosquito vectors.

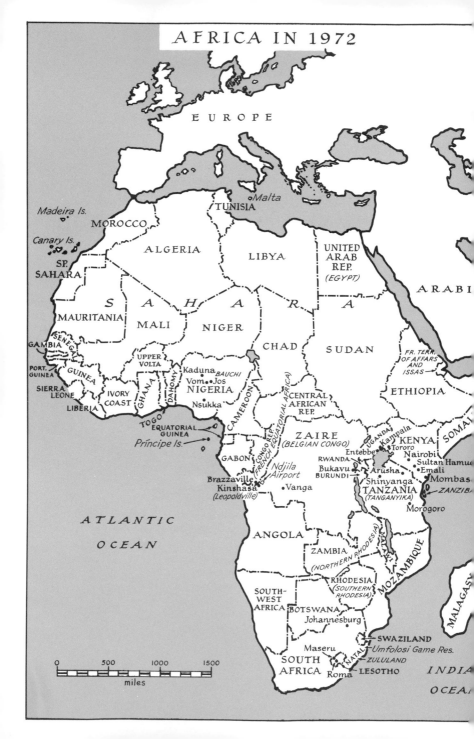

AFRICA IN 1972

EUROPE

Malta

Madeira Is.

MOROCCO

TUNISIA

Canary Is.

ALGERIA

LIBYA

UNITED ARAB REP. (EGYPT)

SP. SAHARA

ARABI

S A H A R A

MAURITANIA

MALI

NIGER

CHAD

SUDAN

FR. TERR. OF AFFARS AND ISSAS

GAMBIA

SENEGAL

UPPER VOLTA

Kaduna *BAUCHI*

ETHIOPIA

PORT. GUINEA

GUINEA

Vom ·· Jos

NIGERIA

CAMEROON

CENTRAL AFRICAN REP.

SIERRA LEONE

IVORY COAST

GHANA

DAHOMY

Nsukka

SOMAI

LIBERIA

TOGO

EQUATORIAL GUINEA

Príncipe Is.

CONGO REP.

FRENCH EQUATORIAL AFRICA

ZAIRE (BELGIAN CONGO)

UGANDA

Kampala

KENYA

Tororo

Entebbe

Nairobi

GABON

Brazzaville

Ndjila Airport

RWANDA

Bukavu

BURUNDI

Arusha

Shinyanga

Sultan Hamud

Emali

Mombas.

Kinshasa (Leopoldville)

· Vanga

TANZANIA (TANGANYIKA)

ZANZIB.

Morogoro

ATLANTIC

OCEAN

ANGOLA

ZAMBIA (NORTHERN RHODESIA)

MOZAMBIQUE

MALAGASY

SOUTH-WEST AFRICA

RHODESIA (SOUTHERN RHODESIA)

BOTSWANA

Johannesburg

SWAZILAND

Umfolosi Game Res.

Maseru

NATAL

ZULULAND

SOUTH AFRICA

Roma

LESOTHO

INDIA

OCEA

| 0 | 500 | 1000 | 1500 |

miles

The growth of the research empire devoted to tsetse and try-panosomes was erratic and kaleidoscopic. Institutionalization of the research and the technology was inevitable as the complexity and the cost of research and action programs mounted. The bureaucracies that were created passed in and out of existence far more readily than one would imagine; they were resilient and responsive to the needs of the people and to the importance of the problem at any one point in time. A devoted general like Richet, who with modest facilities threw all of his energies into action programs for treating people and combating flies, naturally looked with scorn on the construction of splendid research institutes elsewhere. But in their minds if not openly, leaders in those institutes would counter Richet's comment, "The aim pursued is not to carry on research in splendid institutes but to do more urgent work—to prevent men dying," with an equally forceful, "Is that so?" and set about to prove to him and to others that splendid institutes through research could do urgent work to prevent men dying. When the score is tallied, however, the strength and durability of the research-action network will depend upon the combined success of both and upon the African people's assessment of the state of war against tsetse in the light of other great issues which they face.

Health missions, research institutes, and action programs for tsetse fly and sleeping sickness control often blended one into another. In 1875, after France realized the commercial potential of her equatorial African possessions, she sent a mission led by Count Pierre Savorgnan de Brazza to the area of Africa now comprising Chad, the Central African Republic, and the Republic of Congo (Brazzaville). An eminent army doctor, Noël Eugène Ballay, went on that mission and assessed the sleeping sickness problem in the hinterland. Subsequently the Paris Geographical Society and related organizations financed the first scientific medical mission to the Congo (Brazzaville).

Africa in 1972. (Drawn by John Morris.)

De Brazza had become by that time administrator for French Equatorial Africa, but in 1906 another soldier-explorer, Emile Gentil, replaced him. Gentil gave the medical mission "land, a laboratory, and a hospital pavilion" to enable it to build an institute in Brazzaville, which is now the capital of the Republic of the Congo and a sprawling city just a ferryboat ride across Stanley Pool from present-day Kinshasa in Zaire.

In 1908 the Brazzaville institute became one of France's many overseas Pasteur Institutes which, in addition to supporting research, trained young Africans for work with patients suffering from sleeping sickness. In the 1920's, Dr. Eugène Jamot became director of this institute. He developed therefrom his far-flung action program extending throughout French Equatorial Africa.

After Jamot's administration the Brazzaville institute deteriorated and the French deliberated over reconstructing it or intensifying their field campaigns. During this period the Belgians were constructing their splendid new Princess Astride Medical Laboratories at Leopoldville, the colonial name for Kinshasa. Competition was such that the French government then chose to rebuild its institute to surpass the Belgian laboratories in grandeur. Following World War II, the Pasteur Institute at Brazzaville became the equatorial base for World Health Organization activities on sleeping sickness and on other health problems.

One early thrust at international cooperation on problems which the fly brought about went in an unpredictable direction. As long ago as 1907 the British Foreign Office called an international conference to try to devise a common policy and enforceable administrative measures for areas infected or menaced by sleeping sickness. Out of this conference grew the Sleeping Sickness Bureau, which was supposed to be a central agency, international in nature. But various countries concerned could not agree on the necessity for it or on its location, so Lord Elgin, then Secretary of State for the Colonies, established it as a British office, and the Royal Society agreed to house the bureau temporarily in a small ground-floor apartment on its premises. The bureau soon broadened in scope to cover a number of tropical diseases. Four years later, in 1912, it moved to the Imperial Institute and changed its name to Tropical Diseases Bureau, and since then has issued the *Tropical Diseases Bulletin,* an abstracting journal absolutely indispensable to doctors and others who want to keep abreast of the literature on infectious diseases of the tropics. In 1926, with a widened mandate, it was renamed the Bureau of Hygiene and Tropical Diseases.

The Churchillian vision—"International Commissions discuss him round green tables"—gained force as the tsetse fly and sleeping sickness entered into the deliberations in world organizations at the highest level. The ravages of disease on the Russian front during World War I had awakened people to the realization that infectious diseases and medical treatment could no longer remain the haphazard responsibility of private practitioners, mission groups, philanthropic agencies, or even individual nations. Typhus, cholera, relapsing fever, typhoid, dysentery, and smallpox, to name a few, were unwanted international travelers. When the League of Nations was founded in 1920 it therefore created a European Health Committee, which became the League's official Health Organization. It soon extended its scope to include collecting information on sleeping sickness and tuberculosis in equatorial Africa and making recommendations about them.

The Health Organization called two international conferences—one in London in 1925, another in Paris in 1928. Through the London conference it established a working party called the First International Sleeping Sickness Commission, which set up headquarters in Entebbe, Uganda. England, France, Germany, Portugal, and Italy were represented on this commission. It was supposed to exchange information, collate data on clinical conditions of patients, study therapeutic measures for sleeping sickness control, and study the behavior of tsetse. In 1927 the commission turned in an interim report and a year later its final report.

For the control and prevention of sleeping sickness, the Committee recommended: (1) controlling movement of natives from one country to another in sleeping sickness areas, including supplying each person with an identity card as a passport; (2) taking a census of infected natives and keeping that census up to date; (3) compulsory treatment of all cases; (4) removing people from heavily infected zones; and (5) clearing bush, but only in regions where *G. palpalis* was prevalent and where human beings were apt to travel.

When in 1926 the Health Committee of the League of Nations convened for the third time, Dr. L. Raynaud, its leader, reported on the work of its commission on tropical diseases. The commission felt that the League should take an active interest in the fate of the numerous peoples that inhabit Africa. Dr. Raynaud pointed out that not only was the health of the African people the responsibility of the protectors or mandatories but that it was the humanitarian duty of all civilized countries to take account of the spread of sleeping sickness and other infectious diseases, particularly in view of the fact that contact with the white race had without doubt helped transmit the disease outside its original frontiers. He also stressed that although civilization brings advantages it inevitably results in harm as well, and this, he felt, should be made good.

After World War II and the formation of the United Nations, the World Health Organization (WHO) took over and expanded the responsibilities and activities of the League's Health Committee. Sleeping sickness continued to be a disease of concern not only to WHO, but also to the Food and Agricultural Organization (FAO), the United Nations Development Program (UNDP), and the United Nations Educational, Scientific and Cultural Organization (UNESCO).

In addition to supporting the integration of sleeping sickness studies with those of other communicable diseases first in the League and then in the United Nations, the metropolitan powers focused their attention, separately and collectively, on scientific development in Africa generally and on sleeping sickness and tsetse fly in particular.

In 1945 the French and British initiated discussions as to how their governments could communicate and cooperate about programs of science; by 1947 four other powers—the Belgians, the Portuguese, the South Africans, and the Rhodesians—had joined; and by 1950 these six countries together formed the Commission for Technical Cooperation in Africa South of the Sahara (CCTA).

Also, in the mid-forties, the European scientists working in Africa themselves felt a need for a system of cooperation. In London in 1946 the Royal Society held the Empire Scientific Conference, which three years later convened an African regional scientific conference in Johannesburg. Representatives from nearly every country south of the Sahara attended it, and it became the Scientific Council for Africa (CSA). This body worked in the closest association with CCTA from the beginning. It sponsored conferences, symposia, meetings of specialists; it arranged visits and prepared publications. From 1951 to 1954 each organization had an independent secretariat, CSA in Africa and CCTA in London. But at the beginning of 1955 they were amalgamated under a common secretary general; their main office was in London and a small unit worked in Bukavu, the Belgian Congo. One of their most important functions was to organize conferences and meetings on scientific and technical subjects.

In 1948 an Inter-African Conference on Tsetse and Trypanosomiasis was held in Brazzaville in Africa. It recommended that the Bureau Permanent Interafricain pour la Tsé-Tsé et la Trypanosomiase (BPITT) be established for studies on the tsetse fly and trypanosomiasis. The bureau was to be located at Kinshasa (Leopoldville) under joint French and Belgian direction and housed in the new Princess Astride Medical Laboratories. At the same time it recommended the formation of the International Scientific Committee for Trypanosomiasis Research (ISCTR). ISCTR has met nearly every year since then and in 1955 became responsible to CCTA/CSA. In 1965, CCTA became an organ of the Organisation of African Unity, and its functions integrated with those of the Scientific, Technical and Research Commission (STRC). At that time, OAU had thirty-four member states. BPITT was closed down as of 1962.

Vom, Kaduna, Kampala, Nairobi, Brazzaville—one after the other growing metropolises of Africa served as hosts to international conferences, organized by ISCTR, about the tsetse fly and its trypanosomes. These conferences proved to be more than routine paper-reading sessions and job markets. They really brought balance to worldwide research effort; they charted broad attacks on the fly and its diseases through administrative, medical, and entomological control measures; and they gave direction and inspiration to the workers, some of whom came from quite isolated laboratories.

World War II and its aftermath sent tremors through the colonial empires, though a decade passed before changes in political power and new patterns of national boundaries took form. In the late 1940's and early 1950's the brief time left to the colonial powers enabled them to create institutes on African soil that could, as they should, deal with the fly and the diseases broadly over an ecological area irrespective of local boundaries.

In 1945 the Tsetse Fly and Trypanosomiasis Committee of the United Kingdom Colonial Office, itself constituted in 1944, engaged Dr. T. H. Davey, Professor of Tropical Hygiene, School of Medicine, Liverpool University, to examine and report on the whole trypanosomiasis situation of West Africa. He recommended, among other things, the creation of a regional research institute to deal with the problem, and he suggested that the main laboratories be sited in Nigeria because that country had the widest range of climatic conditions that affected the fly and the disease in a compact geographical area. The Nigerian government established the West African Institute for Trypanosomiasis Research (WAITR) in October 1950, with one set of rambling bungalow-style laboratories in the tsetse-fly-infested area around Kaduna and a similar set at Vom near the tin-mining center of Jos in the tsetse-fly-free highland region. The British government met two-thirds of the cost of the initial expenditures; Ghana, Sierra Leone, Gambia, and Nigeria financed the remaining one-third.

The same committee from the United Kingdom felt that much had already been accomplished to eliminate the fly in East Africa but that a great deal more research was necessary on the trypanosomes. The committee deputized Professor Patrick A. Buxton of the London School of Tropical Medicine to tour East Africa, and in 1945 he proposed unifying the several existing branches of research dealing with the fly and the trypanosomes. His recommendations led, in 1946, to the formation of two new organizations—one, the East African Tsetse and Trypanosomiasis Research Organization, the other, the East African Tsetse Reclamation Department. Two years later these two organizations were merged into the East African Trypanosomiasis Research Organization (EATRO) and headquartered in Nairobi, Kenya, until a new unit and central laboratories were constructed at Tororo, high in the hills in Uganda near its eastern border with Kenya. The old Shinyanga and Tinde laboratories of Swynnerton's day and their staffs were included in this new unit. The financial arrangements were similar to those made in West Africa; the Colonial Development and Welfare Fund (CD&W) made a grant for capital construction costs, while the three African territories, Kenya, Tanganyika, and Uganda, put up half of the recurrent costs, which the CD&W matched.

The two new regional institutes—one in West Africa, the other in East Africa—dug into basic research problems. They explored further the ecology of the fly and its great sensitivity to its environment in order that the action programs in Africa could make their insecticide control of tsetse more specific. The research institutes tried to concoct drugs less toxic to animals infected with trypanosomes but more effective against the trypanosomes themselves. And the institutes sampled a whole range of trypanosome species, varieties, and types to find out where the genetic variation in them lay and what this would mean in attempting to manage the trypanosome population so that men and animals could develop tolerance, if not immunity, to it.

The campaigns and similar programs of an action nature to prevent men dying devolved upon individual territories, to the departments of veterinary services and public health in Kenya, Uganda, Tanzania, Nigeria, and others. They did the fieldwork to treat people and to control the fly population, and they accepted what innovations were practical that emanated from the institutes.

Accelerated industrialization, urban growth, an increase in the price of raw materials, creation of a middle class of Africans, improvement in motor traffic, a great increase in the number of schools, an outflow of Africans to other countries, and the growth of a local press—all fueled the revolution of rising expectations among the African population that culminated in independence for one country after another in rapid succession.

First Ghana, then Nigeria, Sierra Leone, and Gambia—the four countries which WAITR served—gained their independence in the late 1950's and early 1960's.

As the political empires crumbled, so did the research empires built on tsetse flies and trypanosomes. New political leadership meant new research leadership. Priorities of research had to be reestablished. The seriousness of sleeping sickness on man and of nagana on cattle had to be reweighed in the context of African peoples' views of more urgent problems. African leadership and an African working force had to be trained rapidly for filling the posts of those going home; laboratory space, equipment needs, and staff housing had to be reassessed; and budgets redrawn. The coming of new life into old institutions could not mean routinely accepting old programs and structures built and being abandoned by other individuals.

In 1962, Director T. A. M. Nash of WAITR, who had pioneered the Anchau Rural Development Scheme, returned to England. He took his flies with him. The Overseas Development Ministry, a successor governmental agency to the Colonial Office, financed the building and support for his home-based laboratory at Bristol. Dr. Nash's deputy, Dr. A. M. Jordan, another medical entomologist, went back to England as one of Nash's colleagues, as he had been at an earlier time in Nigeria. A medical doctor, K. C. Willet, replaced Nash as director of WAITR, but he soon left to join the World Health Organization. Subsequently a veterinarian, Dr. Thomas M. Leach, replaced Willet to hold the institute together during its transition from a regional to a local institution, as it became the Nigerian

Institute for Trypanosomiasis Research (NITR). The institute recently came under the directorship of a young African specialist in trypanosomiasis research, Dr. A. A. Amodu, who received his training in parasitology in the United States. International and regional funding diminished, and local financing from the federal government of Nigeria replaced it. A scramble ensued among young Africans for scholarships that would enable them to become proficient at masters- or doctorate-degree level in various scientific disciplines and for other opportunities to earn their qualifications for scientific and technical posts at NITR and other such institutes.

The East African Trypanosomiasis Research Organization (EATRO) began to undergo wrenches in leadership and in program similar to those at WAITR. Tanzania, Uganda, and Kenya became independent states in the early 1960's. The British High Commission governing Tanzania, Uganda, and Kenya during the 1950's gave way to the East African Common Services Organization, which changed to the East African Community. EATRO weathered the changes and remained under the aegis of the community along with the postal services, the telegraph, the railroads, currency, and customs. During the 1960's, as each nation fashioned its own idealogy and developed its own national identity and pride, the services of the community weakened; each of the nations wished to handle its own affairs. EATRO continued under the community as a regional institute, but as in West Africa the leaders went back home. Dr. W. H. R. Lumsden, the director, who had built the germ-plasm bank of trypanosomes, took up a post at the London School of Medicine and Hygiene. Some of his staff found havens in multilateral international programs dealing with trypanosomiasis, tsetse flies, or other diseases and vectors. An able Ugandan doctor, Dr. R. A. Onyango, took over the leadership of EATRO, and it began to rebuild programs. Leadership has subsequently passed to Dr. A. R. Njogu, a young African immunologist.

The exodus of tsetse and trypanosomiasis workers depleted laboratories in Africa but accelerated basic research on these organisms in the United Kingdom and Europe and stimulated research in Canada and the United States. By the late 1960's research had spread to dozens of foreign laboratories; it was becoming almost a matter of habit, an end in itself rather than a means to an end.

Having spent virtually a lifetime doing research on tsetse flies in Africa, how could Nash, back in Britain, abandon them? He built his laboratory in Bristol primarily to rear tsetse flies to satisfy the research needs of other scientists. He fed his flies on goats and rabbits, usually the former. This was no mean task, for tsetse prefers to select its own food and host. He tried having them feed on cows, but these animals were "too large and too smelly." He employed pigs as a source of food for his flies but they "screamed their heads off," and he finally concluded that goats were the best laboratory animal. Nash allowed his flies to feed fifteen minutes daily except Sunday, one hundred per fifteen-minute period, four hundred in an hour, on four or five goats. And the fly, once the object of scorn and disgust, became hallowed and revered, the object of tender loving care. Soon Nash was exporting flies to laboratories in Lisbon and in other European cities. His success in producing tsetse flies was such that he even gave away thousands of pupae each year. A few years ago production got to the point where his laboratory assistants were killing 17,000 flies a year in order to keep production below 75,000.

In Lisbon, Professor João Fraga de Azevedo, who led the team to eradicate tsetse flies in the early 1950's from Príncipe, developed another colony of tsetse flies. With production rising in both laboratories, and with a fly-rearing laboratory in operation in Paris, flies were pushing people to conduct more research on sleeping sickness. The research followed modern trends, namely basic studies on: the improvement of techniques for rearing tsetse flies en masse so as to make it practical to liberate sterilized male flies to eradicate tsetse flies in nature; the process by which trypanosomes become infective to man and beast after their sojourn in the tsetse salivary glands; the mechanisms by which trypanosomes really do their damage to animals and man; and methods of bringing about immune reactions in man and animals infected by trypanosomes.

But in the mid-1960's the decisive postindependence drive for managing the fly and its trypanosomes had to come from the new nations, from a new constituency, the African people who live in their presence and who have to assess the importance to them of research on these organisms. These new nations have to translate their asessment into financing research and organizing sleeping sickness or cattle trypanosomiasis control programs. They have to decide what to do with the old and where to begin anew.

To renovate the old and to build new physical plants, African planners had to exercise judgment and sensitivity about what to scrap and what to save; they could not operate as archeologists undertaking restorations out of respect for the physical structures of the past. The new research teams that were forming were international ones; equipment, laboratory space, field facilities, and above all modern housing for staff were critically important for the morale and working effectiveness of the team. To Castellani, in 1900–1905, "what shall I wear?" seemed paramount as he thought of the physical conditions he would face in Africa. Today "where shall I live?" looms important.

In one newly organized research program, for example, a former director's spacious colonial home stands idle, maybe because the authority it symbolizes seems inappropriate for the new era, but more likely because it does not meet the demands of modern living for foreigner or African. Blinding white in the Sahara sun and set well back in a parklike area, this two-story house is the largest, most pretentious one. It has an archway veranda extending on either side of the entrance which protects the ground floor rooms from sunlight and excessive heat. Its great foyer, twice the size of dining or living room, was designed for receptions. But the kitchen is antiquated, small and inconveniently arranged. And the wood-planked floors throughout the house, covered with many coats of brown paint, creak. Meanwhile up-to-date ranch-style homes molded to the needs of today's staff have been going up in the same residential area to alleviate a housing shortage.

Spontaneously research efforts on tsetse flies and trypanosomes spring up in the newly created national universities, and these defy the monolithic approach of concentrating all such efforts at one institution in the hands of a few researchers. Several young Nigerian pathologists at the University of Ibadan are attempting to discover how the red blood cells in animals get worried to death by the trypanosomes, a secret that neither Bruce nor anyone who followed him has yet been able to disclose. Another scientist in the University of Rhodesia wants to know how tsetse flies derive a nutritionally balanced meal from the blood they consume, it being largely proteinaceous. At these and other new centers, unencumbered with leftover facilities and residual programs, the investigators have quite the opposite problem from those working in institutions like NITR and EATRO. They must start out in cramped quarters, borrow equipment, and devise ways of cooperating with their colleagues in agriculture or in medicine as well as in animal science.

The growing points of scientific strength in Africa are drawing the attention of international bodies in imaginative ways. In

1970, for example, an International Centre of Research on Insect Physiology and Ecology (ICIPE) was founded in Nairobi, Kenya, and associated with the University of Nairobi. From all over the world, government agencies, philanthropic institutions, academies of science, and universities contributed resources and talent to assist ICIPE in coping with five of East Africa's most important insect pests—tsetse flies, ticks, mosquitoes, army worms, and termites. In addition to a board of directors of international renown, this institute benefits from an international committee which reviews the standards of excellence of the program and the funds required to run it. An African committee performs similar functions and assures that research at ICIPE will be relevant to the pest situation in East Africa. One problem this institute will tackle is the influence that the salivary glands of the fly have upon the virulence of the trypanosomes when they reach the animal host following their passage through these glands in tsetse.

Thomas Odhiambo, ICIPE's research director and one of Africa's leading tsetse scientists, has expressed concern about the ease with which the African nations can accept technology without developing science itself. "The African's monistic (one world) view of nature is an impediment to his becoming a natural scientist," he wrote, and continued:

The most important philosophical concept of the Nilotes' culture is the concept of Jok. Jok can mean three things at the same time: (i) it can mean "the greatest spirit," the great "mover of all things," the creator and sustainer of the world and everything in it, or the equivalent of the Christian idea of God; (ii) it can also mean the spirit, or ghost, or witchcraft, or some form of spiritual power; and (iii) it can also mean the body or matter.

A similar philosophical system is held by the Bantu, who form the preponderant part of the population of Africa south of the Sahara.

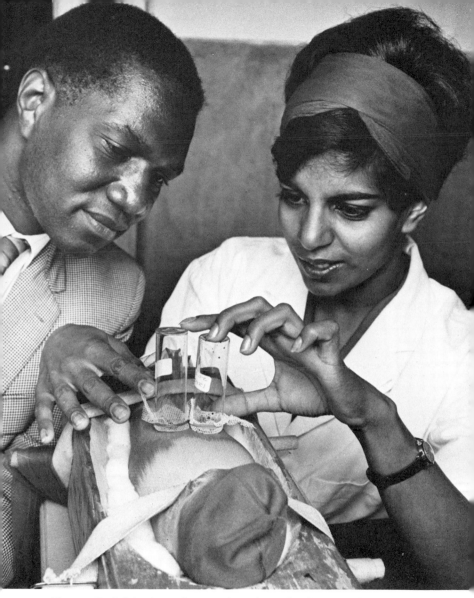

Thomas R. Odhiambo and research assistant feeding flies. (Photograph by Marc & Evelyne Bernheim, from Rapho Guillurmette Pictures by permission of The Rockefeller Foundation.)

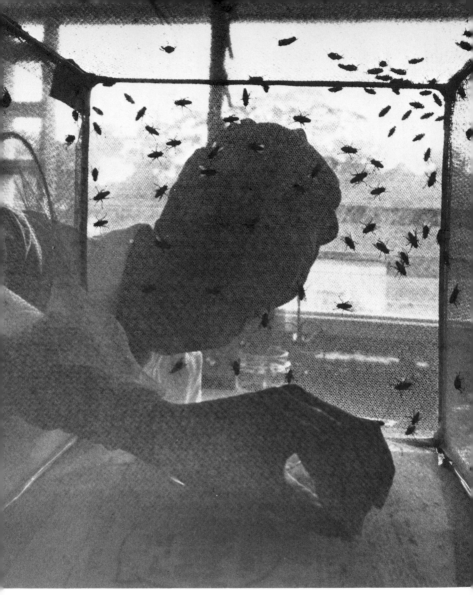

Experimentation with tsetse flies in screen cage. (Photograph by Marc & Evelyne Bernheim, from Rapho Guillurmette Pictures by permission of The Rockefeller Foundation.)

The basic difference between African philosophy and Western philosophy is that the former is based on a concept of being that is dynamic (being is "the force which is"), whereas the latter is static (being is "that which is"). Second, African philosophy is a monism (a one-world view), while Western (and Indian) philosophy is a dualism (a subjective as well as an objective world).

These observations have important consequences for the African's participation in science. In this African philosophy there is no sharp distinction between the subjective and objective worlds, as we find in European and Indian philosophies. In the case of the European, his attempts to make these distinctions have resulted in science; that is, scientists have had to distinguish between belief, faith, taste, and so forth (the subjective world), and the objective impersonal world. In the case of the Indian, his attempts have led him to treat the world as mere appearance (maya); the world exists only in the mind; therefore, there is no objective universe or absolute reality awaiting discovery. Thus, the Indian has mysticism rather than science. As for the African, his monism has deprived him of the choice between either science or mysticism; instead, he has concentrated his intellectual powers in devising a vastly intricate social and communalistic system.

Odhiambo suggests a number of ways in which the African people can prepare themselves and their nations to develop science and ends his article by recalling the words of Malcolm S. Adiseshiah, Deputy Director-General of UNESCO, who, at the closing session of the 1964 Lagos Conference on scientific research, stated that "political independence without scientific knowledge and competence is as contradictory as the concept of a vegetarian tiger."

The early research on tsetse and trypanosomes, the campaigns to control these organisms, and the institutionalization of both research and action programs over the last fifty years have made their impact. For the time being, tsetse is down and out—almost. The trypanosomes which it carries take only a small toll of life among the 328 million human beings on the continent of Africa. In those areas man really cares about, he can and does bring readily under control, and sometimes almost succeeds in eradicating, tsetse and the trypanosomes.

While tsetse and trypanosomes bide their time in the late 1960's and early 1970's, fire burns in the people for education, power, and the right to control their destiny. Archibald Campbell Jordan, a leading South African black poet protesting the injustice of his people's situation voiced their desires and exclaimed: "You tell me to sit quiet."

The insatiable drive for education among Jordan's people now figures as an issue of top priority in southern Africa, where in David Livingstone's time combating a fly that attacked their cattle seemed paramount. Against unbelievable odds the countries of Lesotho, Botswana, and Swaziland, for example, are building a university, though they share no common boundary, have no common ethnic background, and must depend on sources outside the borders of their countries for financial support for the university. Situated in Lesotho three steep gorges beyond Maseru, its capital, the University of Botswana, Lesotho, and Swaziland (UBLS) struggles to impart knowledge in basic sciences to a small body of students on the main campus; its branch in Swaziland trains young men in agriculture; and its outpost in Botswana gives instruction to students in animal husbandry.

At UBLS the ghost appears of a tsetse and trypanosome fighter of long ago. When I was invited to the vice chancellor's home in 1966, I saw in the dining room a photograph of a grave and a gravestone in the Antrim Hills of Ireland, the vice chancellor's country. Taken some thirty years ago, it portrays a setting (or rising) sun behind a cross of stone which the corona of the hidden sun outlines brilliantly. It is a dramatic picture of the former grave of Sir Roger Casement, who was reinterred with honors in Ireland's National Cemetery in 1965. It is appropriate that this picture should have been carried to Africa near Swaziland and Natal, where Casement once lived and worked; sixty years earlier he had done much to *educate* people as to the importance of sleeping sickness and had given impetus to the studies that ensued on the relationship of this disease to tsetse.

Tsetse and sleeping sickness problems seem to have ebbed in Zaire, where in colonial days Casement made his greatest impact. Long after Stanley, Glave, and Casement were dead, the Belgians turned the fly-infested high-grass savanna area along the east bank of Stanley Pool into a modern landing field and airport. They brought in heavy equipment and large quantities of insecticide which they applied liberally to eradicate tsetse flies from this area. They built the airport without losing a single laborer to sleeping sickness. Today one may travel by Air Zaire, Sabena, Pan American, and other airlines, land at Ndjila International Airport (its present name) near Kinshasa and encounter few, if any, flies, and those, most likely, not of the tsetse variety. Or he may ferry across the Congo River at Stanley Pool where the clumps of water hyacinths race each other to the cataracts; scarcely a tsetse will be there to bite.

In Zaire, a restless nation with a positive outlook, the people seek "autenticité" and address themselves to their educational needs with vigor. On a bluff overlooking Stanley Pool and the city of Kinshasa stands the main campus of the Université Nationale de Zaire (UNAZA). One of the tributaries of the Congo River, the Ndjila, which flows along the north side of Kinshasa cuts between the campus and the university's experimental grounds. This university houses a nuclear reactor, operates a first-class medical school and teaching hospital, and offers instruction in the basic sciences and agriculture geared to colonial interests in the past. The university is now in the throes of a reorganization in order that its course work and research will reflect Zaire's needs. The state of war against tsetse as the Zairois assess it will dictate the role that this institution may play in further research and action programs to keep tsetse and its trypanosomes subdued.

Deep in Zaire, in the Congo of old that Glave pictured, the outlook is now one of optimism from people less encumbered with disease and oppression than formerly. The curse has been lifted, and one can witness the emergence of leadership and power that for nation building must come from all occupations and all levels of educational achievement. At a religious mission station situated at Vanga in abandoned oil-palm country on the Kwilu River, a tributary of the Congo, activity at the wharf is no longer lethargic, but vital. A gangplank connects a freighter to a truck. On this plank rests a tremendous crate bowing it to the cracking point. In this humid and sweaty place a group of men dressed in shorts and singlets with bare feet crowd upon the splintery plank to move the crate, but they can neither push nor pull it. Spontaneously help comes as someone from the group begins to chant a work song. All respond, and a leader is born. Muscles and tendons tighten and relax to a rhythm. From ship to truck, inch by inch, the crate moves down the plank to the cadence of a song.

In Kenya lies Nairobi, a highland city which probably never suffered the scourge of tsetse fly or sleeping sickness. This city was once just a railroad yard; then a stopover village for such men as Lord Lugard, the Cook brothers, Sir Winston Churchill, and many others on their way from Mombasa to the Lake Victoria port towns of Uganda; subsequently a gateway to the so-called white or European highlands of colonial days.

Social and political problems seem far more acute in Nairobi than does fighting tsetse. In fact, disagreeable domestic insects command attention that might better go to tsetse. In

1965 an Indian technician who worked for the professor of botany at University College, Nairobi (now the University of Nairobi), invited her professor and me home for tea. She, her huszand, and small child lived on the east side of town close to the game park in a two-story home of cement construction with casement windows. Her husband, an Asian doctor refugee from Pakistan at the time of partition, had barely escaped that country with his life. He subsequently studied in the United States and the United Kingdom and finally moved to Nairobi, where, despite Asian and European discrimination, he developed a lucrative practice. Naturally, conversation among Indian technician, Asian doctor, African scientist, and American visitor turned to the stability of the governments of East Africa and to the prospects members of minority groups might have for jobs and security. In the dining area the doctor's wife served cookies and cakes. The sun shining through the window warmed excessively the young African botanist's back. He turned and flicked the curtains across the window. A cloud of cockroaches of all sizes came down from the valance and scampered across the table for cover. They turned the overheated discussion on discrimination to a thoughtful conversation of what insecticides might most effectively control these pests.

With or without the scourge of tsetse directly upon it and despite the attention lesser insects may attract, Nairobi through its university and government offices is destined to play a critical role in determining what research will receive support and what reclamation programs need to be implemented to wrest land from tsetse where it survives and in some cases prospers. The growth and development of the University of Nairobi, on whose grounds the International Centre of Insect Physiology and Ecology (ICIPE) is built and from whose student body and staff ICIPE draws talent for research on tsetse flies, will influence that of ICIPE. Financial and policy backing that the veterinary services receive from the Kenya government will determine the extent to which field programs and research can free areas of the country from the fly. Kenya's posture toward the East African Community, like that of Tanzania and Uganda, will affect the strength and the scope of research done by the East African Trypanosomiasis Research Organization (EATRO) at Tororo on tsetse flies and on trypanosomiasis over East Africa as a whole.

Beyond Nairobi in the lowland game country where tsetse thrives, people move around less fearful than formerly of tsetse and of their own inadequacies in coping with the African bush. The lion is tamed, or at least tamable; it comes to people to have them brush tsetse from its back. Joy Adamson of *Born Free* fame welcomed the lion for the deflying function she could perform. In this instance tsetse became a tool in the hands of an expert who turned it to advantage in establishing and maintaining a "peek-a-boo" relationship with the wild beasts of Africa and with the Africa of the past.

Population pressures of human beings hungry for cleared land pitted against those of the fly to keep cattle and people away indicate that human beings may be winning in Morogoro, Tanzania. In clearing the land of this beautiful valley the people have left hardly any room for the fly; large sisal plantations occupy the rolling lowlands. Construction of an agricultural school began in the foothills of this valley in the early 1960's; it soon became the agricultural faculty of the University of Dar es Salaam. Africans and Asians reside in Morogoro, while European expatriates live in isolated luxury on the hillsides surrounding it.

The stresses and strains associated with Africanization seem further to relegate tsetse to insignificance in this area, once under Swynnerton's tsetse control campaign. In 1965 their personal concerns, the realization, for example, that Africans would soon replace them, were the topic of expatriate conversation, not tsetse. On the slopes of one of these hills lived a handsome redheaded expatriate, director of the land planning institute associated with the college. As we sat on the veranda of his home on a bright sunny day we heard the crush of gravel and saw a Volkswagen appear in the driveway. An English woman dressed in a faded steel-gray uniform alighted. She sold Girl Guide badges to the scattered families in Tanzania, who in turn parceled out the awards to their daughters as they completed their requirements. Both enjoyed their occupations and expressed keen regret that local persons might replace them.

Throughout Africa a whole generation of youths of different ages with varying degrees of education and technical skills are preparing to fill the gap present workers leave as they, for whatever reason, move to other posts. In West Africa years have passed since WAITR became NITR. Tsetse still feeds in the wild; people still contract sleeping sickness. Man's mastery of tsetse will depend on a new corps of workers. Among them young boys will be just as essential to the success of the research as were those a generation ago, and research needs will open up opportunities for them to become the career investigators of the future.

Within the working range of NITR in the northern part of Nigeria, for instance, a boy comes to the river's edge to draw water. He is lucky to be in the outdoors and to have the riverbank as his gymnasium and a man-sized bucket of water for his set of dumbbells. He builds his biceps by straining to lift the brimfull pail to his head. The weight of the water helps him to straighten his back. His unsteady gait brings down splashes of water to cool his shoulders and to lighten his load. Proud to have worked up to being able to carry such a heavy burden, he picks his way along a narrow dirt path into bush where wheelbarrow or cart would be of little use. As he grows up, will this young boy roll over the logs to look underneath them for the tsetse pupae which might be there? Will he arrange these logs in order to make a bait environment where tsetse flies can deposit their larvae? If he eventually works for NITR, it will not be at sixpence a day as did Nash's fly boys years ago. Almost certainly he will go forth with a Geiger counter to seek tsetse flies marked with radioactive cobalt and to record where they may be hiding.

Man may think he is lord and master of the tsetse flies. But is he really? Dr. Evans D. Offori, a Ghanaian who has been with the International Atomic Energy Agency in Vienna undertaking studies on the irradiation technique of sterilizing male tsetse flies, might caution in his own language, Ewe: "Vu mevona le adzoe fe ta me o. [You will always find blood in the head of a tsetse fly.] We normally crush it by squeezing the head," he adds. The proverb means that a veteran like tsetse always has something up his sleeve.

Time may be on the side of tsetse in West Africa. Nsukka, a town in the eastern part of Nigeria, has been populated with tsetse flies since time immemorial, though sleeping sickness in man and nagana in cattle are under reasonable control in that area today. Nsukka became the home of a new university, the University of Nigeria, in 1962. The agricultural faculty had cleared part of the five thousand acres of land it controlled for an experimental farm. Here the animal husbandmen of the faculty had corralled a number of white Fulani cattle behind a barbed wire enclosure on a hill. Occasionally, a white Fulani cow contracted trypanosomiasis. First she went "off her feed," then sulked in a corner. Her head went down, her ears drooped, and her temperature rose. A veterinarian took her temperature and injected her with the appropriate drug to combat the trypanosomes.

Tsetse flies were not the only insects in this area. While

watching the corralled cattle, one had to be careful not to rest
an elbow on the wrong strand of the barbed wire, for soldier
ants that bite severely marched along certain strands of wire.
When the rains begin, scads of delicate gray, golden-winged termites swarm about; they outnumber tsetse. Schoolchildren catch
and eat these termites. Bigger brown ones collect at the house
lights in the evening. Bluebottle flies buzz around, though like
tsetse not in great numbers. Cows in the corral depended to
some extent upon the egrets (white herons) which follow them
to help clean up all these flies.

In 1967 the area around Nsukka unfortunately became a
frontier that both Nigerians and secessionist Biafrans claimed
as theirs for ethnic, economic, and political reasons which
seemed far more serious than pursuing research and control
measures on the fly. This war, which ended in 1970, exposed
the eastern part of Nigeria briefly to a classic danger that Harold Oldroyd warned about, in his *Natural History of Flies,*
when he characterized tsetse as a spectacular relict among those
flies about to drop off the evolutionary ladder:

Although they fight back and win local victories, they will eventually lose, provided that the African continent becomes agricul-
turally and industrially developed like the rest of the world. If, for
political reasons, there should be a temporary reversal of this trend,
then tsetse, and other biting flies too, will get a new lease of life.

Fortunately, thus far tsetse seems not to have responded in a
major way to the opportunity the war-torn eastern part of Nigeria afforded it to make Oldroyd's prophecy come true.

Enforced contact with the fly is still on tsetse's side; it happens throughout Africa today as it always has in the past.
Amidst fishermen, launderers, and bystanders, a young woman
goes down by the water's edge along the Njala River in Sierra
Leone, for example. She does not come from an antiseptic ham-

let or city. She flaunts fate even further, disrobes and exposes herself to all sorts of -arias and -iases as she plunges into the river—to a variety of forms of malaria, schistosomiasis, onchocerciasis, filariasis, and trypanosomiasis, each with its special vector waiting. She and the vectors of these diseases may have no other source of water. In that habitat, tell tsetse to sit quiet, not to bite? In Jordan's words:

> Tell the winter not to give birth to spring.
> Tell the spring not to flower into summer.

In fact, one can imagine tsetse contemptuously posing Jordan's remark as a question to its inattentive host and human enemy: "You tell *me* to sit quiet?"

Uganda, that beautiful garden of death which bore the brunt of the sleeping sickness epidemic at the turn of the century, did indeed spring to life and fulfill Winston Churchill's early impression of that country as a fairy tale. The lake shores that Sir Hesketh Bell depopulated in the early 1900's in order to separate people from tsetse flies now enjoy a prosperous agriculture, evident from the fragrance that comes from the white starlike blossoms of the ubiquitous coffee bush and from the deep green color of orderly, well-cultivated tea plantations. Africans, Indians, Europeans, and other ethnic groups contribute style and variety to life in Kampala, Entebbe, and other shore-line cities; Makerere University, not far from Sir Albert Cook's hospital on Mengo Hill, overlooks the town and adds an aura of sophistication to the city. Research on tsetse is under way at the laboratories at Makerere. Several investigators are conducting feeding trials; they use pedigreed tsetse flies imported from Nash's laboratories in Bristol, England.

Again, not all is as beautiful as it may seem; people have been inattentive. That fertile area which Sir Hesketh Bell worked so hard to free of sleeping sickness did not remain depopulated, as it was until 1920. Endowed with a well-distributed rainfall pattern of forty-five to fifty inches a year, this area grew into thicket and dense forest rapidly and luxuriantly; it afforded ideal cover under which bush buck, bush pig, and the thicket tsetse, *Glossina pallidipes,* could prosper. Stragglers from the migrations of other peoples throughout the eastern part of Uganda began to populate this shore region. Originally pastoralists, they could not maintain the remnants of their herds of cattle, sheep, and goats in this area once again dominated by tsetse, so they exploited these shorelines rich in game by exercising their prowess in hunting and fishing to earn a living.

By the early 1940's sleeping sickness broke out a second time in epidemic proportions in Busoga, the site of the original epidemic in the early 1900's. Authorities reported 2,432 cases of disease, 274 deaths. Probably laborers—9,000 of whom had recently been brought to the area to work on sugar estates which bordered the lake by the town of Jinja— introduced the disease, this time caused by *Trypanosoma rhodesiense* and transmitted by *G. pallidipes.* Resettlement on a grand scale of these people who had moved into the *pallidipes* thicket belt was contemplated and partially implemented, but the scheme failed for the same reasons that contributed to earlier failures—lack of appreciation of many factors of human psychology and sociology. The people did not like being moved from the places where they chose to live and die. Resettlement continued in unorganized and haphazard fashion, and in the early 1970's over two hundred new cases of sleeping sickness a year were being contracted in the area. Tell tsetse with its trypanosomes to sit quiet? As Archibald Campbell Jordan said:

> Go tell the drooping grass,
> Frost-bitten and pale,
> Not to quicken when roused
> By the warm summer rains.

Tsetse, relict from the past, is fighting back. An article in the *New York Times* suggests that people have been overconfident: "W. T. Davis, Diplomat, Fights Disease that Claimed Wife." A former United States ambassador to Switzerland and his wife had gone on safari to the lion country in East Africa in the summer of 1969. Tsetse must have bitten them there and infected them with sleeping sickness. In 1972 two patients were diagnosed and treated for sleeping sickness in Canada. One was a twenty-seven-year-old Caucasian woman who as a volunteer had taught for two years in a mission school in Zaire. The other was a twenty-four-year-old man who had worked for a year as a biologist in a tsetse-fly-infested area of Tanzania. His case, diagnosed first in a mission hospital, showed cerebral involvement. When treated with Mel B, he suffered a severe reaction and was flown to Canada for the management of his condition.

To be complacent about tsetse is indeed to tempt fate, to paint a glorious picture on a canvas subject to insect infestation —as some artists in Kinshasa have to do who, for want of better material, paint on wheat sacks that come from abroad which are permeated with flour that the flour beetles like. In Zaire, after the incidence of sleeping sickness had fallen to rock bottom at a tenth of one per cent of the total population in 1960, it rose. By 1966 forty times as many people contracted the disease as had six years earlier. In some areas 14 per cent of the people caught the disease. Tsetse still prevents cattle being used as beasts of burden in tropical Zaire; the job on tsetse remains to be done. In Ethiopia sleeping sickness is not known to have occurred until 1967, when four cases were confirmed. Twenty-eight cases were diagnosed in 1968, one hundred and seventy-three in 1969, and forty-two in the first ten months of 1970—all along the Gilo River in the southwestern part of the country, Ilubabor province.

What does the future portend? Only a handful of tsetse flies need to survive to generate waves of disease, sickness, and death such as have occurred time and again in years gone by. Tsetse has already given every indication of an invincible capacity to survive, even to thrive. Tsetse, if it has to, may adapt to modern African environments, find domestic niches, and retaliate. One worker, Dr. D. A. T. Baldry, looking for *G. tachinoides* near the city of Nsukka, did not find the puparia of this species in the classical breeding sites around bushy riverbanks. He found them instead in loose soil beneath the overhanging eaves of a house, in soil under a pile of cocoyam tubers, at the base of the spaces between the slats of a fence around a pigpen; and under water storage urns just outside the fence.

It is not possible to lift completely the curse that flies inflict on people, to close the book on tsetse, one of "the special pets of the Creator," which must be divine, certainly not a "bug" in the ordinary sense. Tell tsetse to sit quiet? Nonsense! *

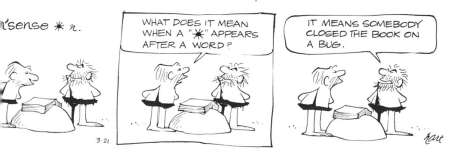

Asterisks and bugs, "B.C." cartoon. (By permission of John Hart and Field Enterprises, Inc.)

The persistent need to keep tsetse down and out—almost—must be heeded. To prevent men dying from sleeping sickness and to open up parts of tropical Africa to the use of cattle as beasts of burden and as a source of protein to feed hungry people constitute essential goals today. To attain them will require competent field staff versed in all the modern techniques for combating tsetse and teams of research workers in institutes probing for further information on the vulnerability of the fly and of trypanosomes.

Bibliographical Essay
and Chapter Notes

GENERAL WORKS

To understand fully the impact tsetse flies have had upon the lives of the people in Africa, one should read widely in the literature of a general nature about Africa, entomology, tsetse flies, and the trypanosomes that cause sleeping sickness in man and nagana in cattle.

Africa

Books about Africa have formed a notable part of the publishing explosion in the last few years, but the appearance since 1960 of many new works of the first rank has not eclipsed the best of the older ones; the most useful are mentioned here and in the chapter notes.

John Gunther's *Inside Africa* (New York: Harper, 1955) provides a fairly accurate general introduction to Africa as it was about 1950. *Africa: A Handbook to the Continent,* edited by Colin Legum, and published in two editions, the first in 1962, the revised in 1966, by Frederick A. Praeger, New York, has short essays on various topics relating to the continent as a whole, as well as a section on each country.

Lord Malcolm Hailey's mammoth undertaking, *An African Sur-*

vey, Revised 1956 (London and New York: Oxford University Press, 1957), successor to a 1938 work, is an invaluable source of information on almost anything concerning the continent at the end of the colonial period. George H. T. Kimble's two-volume *Tropical Africa* (New York: Twentieth Century Fund, 1960) is geographical and sociopolitical in its orientation, more readable and perhaps more provocative than the Hailey. An updated version by George H. T. Kimble and Ronald Steel was published under the title *Tropical Africa Today* (St. Louis: Webster, 1966).

The African World: A Survey of Social Research, edited by Robert A. Lystad for the African Studies Association (New York: Frederick A. Praeger, 1965), is a symposium volume in which the contributions describe the development and status during the early 1960's of various disciplines as they related to Africa. Edgar B. Worthington's *Science in the Development of Africa* (London: CCTA/CSA, 1958) provides extensive background on the role played by the physical as well as by the life sciences; it features a fifteen-page bibliography which includes many journal articles.

The various works by Basil Davidson provide a good introduction to African history—perhaps because of his obvious enthusiasm for the continent and its people. *African Kingdoms* (New York: Time Inc., 1966) from the Time-Life series "Great Ages of Man" presents a delightful panoramic treatment of African history, and Davidson's *The African Past: Chronicles from Antiquity to Modern Times* (Boston: Little, Brown, 1964) brings together a wealth of information from other works by distinguished scholars of African history. Among the histories, one with an especially good bibliography is Robert I. Rotberg, *A Political History of Tropical Africa* (New York: Harcourt, Brace and World, 1965). In paperback, there is a standard work by Roland Oliver and J. D. Fage, *A Short History of Africa* (Baltimore: Penguin Books, 1962). Both these distinguished British scholars have also produced various other works in African history, separately and together. A recent addition to the comprehensive histories of Africa is Robert W. July's *A History of the African People* (New York: Charles Scribner's Sons, 1970).

A welcome trend in African historiography is the increasing number of works being published by scholars who are themselves African. Three well-regarded general ones are: J. F. Ade Ajayi and Ian Espie, eds., *A Thousand Years of West African History* (Ibadan: Ibadan University Press, 1965; New York: Humanities Press, 1965, 2d ed., 1967, 1969); A. Adu Boahen, *Topics in West African History* (New York; Humanities Press, 1966), and B. A. Ogot and J. A. Kieran, eds., *Zamani: A Survey of East African History* (New York: Humanities Press, 1968, 1971). The first and third include essays by both Africans and Europeans.

Two rewarding but somewhat more difficult works are Daniel F. McCall, *Africa in Time-Perspective: A Discussion of Historical Reconstruction from Unwritten Sources* (Boston: Boston University Press, 1964; Legon: Ghana University Press, 1964), and George P. Murdock, *Africa: Its Peoples and Their Culture History* (New York: McGraw-Hill, 1959). The latter is essentially a compendium of ethnographic data, covering both general topics and cultural regions, but it has a historical approach.

A fascinating monograph on a special topic is Philip D. Curtin's *The Image of Africa: British Ideas and Action, 1780–1850* (Madison: University of Wisconsin Press, 1964). Also recommended for the general reader are the books by the noted British soldier-businessman, E. W. Bovill: *Caravans of the Old Sahara* (London: Oxford University Press, 1933) and *The Golden Trade of the Moors* (London: Oxford University Press, 1958; 2d ed., 1968).

The most comprehensive source of purely ethnographic information on Africa and its people—at least in English—is the monograph series entitled *Ethnographic Survey of Africa,* which has been appearing under the editorship of Daryll Forde and the sponsorship of the International African Institute, London, since 1950.

Two especially useful works in economic geography are William A. Hance, *The Geography of Modern Africa* (New York: Columbia University Press, 1964) and L. Dudley Stamp, *Africa: A Study in Tropical Development* (New York: John Wiley, 1953; London: Chapman and Hall, 1953).

Among the atlases, I have found Volume IV: *Southern Europe and Africa* of *The Times Atlas of the World: Mid-Century Edition,* edited by John Bartholomew (London: Times, 1956) the most useful. A one-volume comprehensive edition of *The Times Atlas of the World* (Boston: Houghton Mifflin, 1967; London: Times, 1967) contains the same maps brought up to date. Offering less geographic detail, but with a large range of special maps, is the *Oxford Regional Economic Atlas: Africa,* prepared by P. H. Ady (Oxford: Clarendon Press, 1965). For those who want to read extensively in African history, John D. Fage's *An Atlas of African History* (New York: St. Martin's, 1958; London: Edward Arnold, 1958) is virtually indispensable; however, a new edition is needed.

Copiously illustrated books about Africa form a special category. The one I like best is Leslie Brown's *Africa: A Natural History* (New York: Random House, 1965). Especially on East Africa, Peter Hill Beard's *The End of the Game* (New York: Viking, 1965) is as notable for the drawings as the photographs. In a volume with a dual title Peter Matthiessen is the author of the text *The Tree Where Man Was Born* and Eliot Porter is the photographer of fine color photographs of people, animals, and terrain portraying vividly *The African Experience,* especially in the Sudan and East Africa (New York: E. P. Dutton, 1972).

Many journals could be mentioned. *African Abstracts* includes historical and ethnographic material not readily found in medical and entomological sources. *Africa Report* provides current coverage of the continent; and the *Journal of African History* is the senior serial publication in that discipline.

Entomology

General information about entomology and its practitioners in past times may be found in George H. Carpenter's article "Entomology," in the *Encyclopaedia Britannica,* 11th ed. (1911); in L. O. Howard, *A History of Applied Entomology (Somewhat Anecdotal)* (Washington, D.C.: Smithsonian Institution, 1930; Smithsonian Miscellaneous Collections, Vol. 84), and in parts of E. O. Essig, *A History of Entomology* (New York: Macmillan, 1931).

Several good books for the general reader interested in entomology became available while this book was in preparation. Harold Oldroyd of the British Museum (Natural History) is the author of the useful and interesting *The Natural History of Flies* (New York: Norton, 1965). Marcel Leclercq's *Entomological Parasitology: The Relations between Entomology and the Medical Sciences*, translated by C. Lapage (Oxford and New York: Pergamon Press, 1969), is difficult, but helpful. In a lighter vein are Howard Ensign Evans' excellent *Life on a Little-Known Planet* (New York: E. P. Dutton, 1968), Brian Hocking's *Six-Legged Science* (Cambridge, Mass.: Schenkman, 1968), and Vincent Dethier's earlier *To Know a Fly* (San Francisco: Holden-Day, 1963), a highly personal account of his work with the black blowfly.

Tsetse Flies

Ernest Edward Austen's *A Monograph of the Tsetse-Flies (Genus Glossina, Westwood), Based on the Collection in the British Museum* (London: British Museum (Natural History), 1903; facsimile reprint, New York: Johnson Reprint, 1966), with its many historical notes, remains, after more than half a century, one of the most fascinating books ever written on the subject. Austen also wrote *A Handbook of the Tsetse-Flies* (London: British Museum (Natural History), 1911). Other classical works on tsetse include E. E. Austen and Emile Hegh, *Tsetse-Flies, Their Characteristics, Distribution and Bionomics* (London: Imperial Bureau of Entomology, 1922); Hegh's *Les Tsétsés* (Brussels: Imprimerie Industrielle et Financière (Société Anonyme), 1929; Ministère des Colonies, Royaume de Belgique); R. Newstead, *Guide to the Study of Tsetse-Flies*, written with Alwen R. Evans and W. H. Potts (London: Hodder and Stoughton, 1924; Liverpool School of Tropical Medicine Memoir, new series, No. 1); and C. F. M. Swynnerton's monumental volume *The Tsetse Flies of East Africa: A First Study of Their Ecology, with a View to Their Control* (London: Royal Entomological Society, 1936; *Transactions of the Royal Entomological Society of London*, Vol. 84).

Important works of more recent vintage are Patrick A. Buxton's comprehensive *The Natural History of Tsetse Flies* (London: H. K. Lewis, 1955; London School of Hygiene and Tropical Medicine, Memoir No. 10) and J. P. Glasgow's *The Distribution and Abundance of Tsetse* (New York: Macmillan, distributing for Pergamon Press, Oxford, 1963); Glasgow updated this book with his article entitled "Recent fundamental work on tsetse flies," *Annual Review of Entomology* 12: 421–438, 1967. T. A. M. Nash, one of whose projects in Nigeria is discussed in Chapter III, is the author of *Africa's Bane: The Tsetse Fly* (London: Collins, 1969). John Ford has written a 568-page text on *The Role of the Trypanosomiases in African Ecology: A Study of the Tsetse Fly Problem* (Oxford: Clarendon Press, 1971). This book covers his career dealing with tsetse fly and trypanosomiasis problems in the five countries of Africa in which he has worked: Nigeria, Rhodesia, Uganda, Tanzania, and Kenya.

Many studies containing basic information on tsetse, but more restricted than the above by geographical coverage or other characteristics, are, of course, available, and some of them will be referred to below.

Sleeping Sickness

A wealth of material is available about sleeping sickness. The works that I found most useful for my own understanding include the treatments in Henry Harold Scott's two-volume *A History of Tropical Medicine* (London: Edward Arnold, 1939; Baltimore: Williams and Wilkins, 1939; a second edition was published by both companies in 1942); Charles Wilcocks' *Aspects of Medical Investigation in Africa* (London and New York: Oxford University Press, 1962); and T. A. M. Nash's "A Review of the African trypanosomiasis problem," *Tropical Diseases Bulletin* 57 (10):973–1003, October 1960. The most comprehensive modern compendium of the trypanosomiases and their vectors in Africa is *The African Trypanosomiases*, edited by H. W. Mulligan (New York: John Wiley, 1970), which, heavily oriented toward the British research work, is a prime source of reference. Preceding Part I of this book, which embodies highly technical material, A. J. Duggan presents (pp. xli–lxxxviii) an extremely readable historical perspective of the research and the control programs that developed on tsetse flies and on trypanosomes causing sleeping sickness and nagana. I would recommend it as a comparative analysis with the historical perspective I have presented herein.

A word should be said about American trypanosomiasis, although the vector—a cone-nosed reduvid bug—bears no relationship to tsetse. American trypanosomiasis, or Chagas' disease, is treated in the Scott volume mentioned above, and in a recent WHO publication, *Comparative Studies of American and African Trypanosomiasis* (Geneva, 1969; World Health Organization Technical Report Series, No. 411) as well as in many other sources.

The professional abstracting journal which I as an entomologist studying tsetse have found most helpful is *Tropical Diseases Bulletin*. It reviews and abstracts recent books and articles about both African and American trypanosomiasis and gives a yearly summary of published material on these diseases each May. The *Review of Applied Entomology, Series B; Medical and Veterinary* is another abstracting source of a general nature on tsetse flies and trypanosomes. The *Bulletin of Entomological Research* was the most fruitful of the professional economic and medical entomology journals.

Chapter Notes

—Each section of the notes below refers to a division within the chapter in question.

CHAPTER I—THE CURSE OF FLIES

Pages 1–7

The quotation heading the chapter comes from Mark Twain's long-suppressed *Letters from the Earth* (New York: Harper and Row, 1962), Letter Seven, page 31. It sets one underlying theme which persists throughout this book—the nature of pestilence and disease as a curse from above, therefore divine and not eradicable.

Teff thrives as a cereal crop at altitudes in Ethiopia generally higher than those at which wheat does well. Teff is a minuscule seeded "love grass," which, viewed from a distance, could be mistaken for wheat as the winds play over the fields and generate waves among its panicles. Ground into flour and baked as Mexicans bake tortillas, it turns out as a soft, unleavened "bread" with a pleasantly sour taste. Cooked in this way, Ethiopians call it *injera* and use it as a base for *wat*, a hotly seasoned stew.

Harold Oldroyd refers to the use of smoldering masses of rope to ward off black flies in his *The Natural History of Flies* (New York: Norton, 1965), pp. 66–67.

T. A. M. Nash in *Africa's Bane* (1969) and Edward W. Bovill in *The Golden Trade of the Moors* (1968) provide source material for the speculations about sleeping sickness and nagana in West Africa centuries ago. Nehemiah Levtzion has written an article on "The thirteenth- and fourteenth-century kings of Mali," *Journal of African History* 4 (3): 341–353, 1963.

The reference to Doalu Bukere comes from Sir Harry Johnston's two-volume work on *Liberia* (London: Hutchinson, 1906), I: 230; II: 1107–1114. Those who want to pursue the subject further may wish to read P. E. H. Hair, "Notes on the discovery of the Vai script, with a bibliography," *Sierra Leone Language Review* 2: 36–49, 1963.

Akin L. Mabogunje, a brilliant African geographer at the University of Ibadan, tells in several of his publications about the founding of that city, one of the few large cities of modern Africa that maintain an overwhelmingly African character in layout and in activity. See his account "Ibadan—Black Metropolis," *Nigeria Magazine* No. 68: 15–26, March 1961, and "The growth of residential districts in Ibadan," *Geographical Review* 52: 56–77, 1962.

Pages 7–8

The edition of John Atkins' *The Navy-Surgeon: or, a Practical System of Surgery*, whose Appendix, page 18, is quoted, was published in London in 1734, but apparently there was a 1732 edition.

Pages 8–13

The quest for specific knowledge as to who caught the type specimen *Glossina palpalis,* the most important tsetse that transmits sleeping sickness, led me down many luxuriant garden paths, but this point, as far as I know, remains secret. The search took me to accounts of some fabulous expeditions; notable among these was the sad story, highly readable, of the Tuckey adventure as presented in his *Narrative of an Expedition to Explore the River Zaire, Usually Called the Congo, in South Africa, in 1816, under the Direction of Captain J. K. Tuckey, R.N. . . . .* (London: John Murray, 1818; reprinted London: Cass, 1967). The Introduction to this volume is the source of several quotations: those about John Cranch come from pages lxxii and lxxvi, the reference to Cook's third voyage, attributed to Dr. Douglas, is from its first two pages, and that describing the cause of death is found on page xliii. Its Appendix No. IV, page 418, provided the information that only thirty-six species reached England; the lack of insects was noted on page 357 in a section of "General Observations."

My search also exposed some of the eccentricities of early entomologists, among them Count Dejean as reported in statements quoted from L. O. Howard's *A History of Applied Entomology (Somewhat Anecdotal)* (Washington, D.C.: Smithsonian Institution, 1930), p. 206. A Dr. Boisduval contributed a long obituary entitled "Notice sur M. le Comte Dejean" to *Annales de la société entomologique de France,* 2d ser., III: 499–520, 1845.

André Jean Baptiste Robineau-Desvoidy's *Essai sur les Myodaires* (Paris, 1830; Mémoires présentés par divers Savans a l'Académie Royale des Sciences de l'Institut de France . . . Sciences Mathématiques et Physiques, Tome deuxième) illustrates the thought of the time when one referred to Myodaria as a subsection within the then suborder Diptera, and when among the Myodaria were included the Muscoidea, the houseflies and the tsetse flies. See Charles H. T. Townsend's twelve-part *Manual of Myiology* (Itaquaquecetuba, São Paulo, Brazil: Charles Townsend, 1934–1942), Part 2 (1935): 86–87 and 105–117. C. R. W. Wiedemann figured among the first to describe tsetse in his *Aussereuropaische zweiflü-gelige Insekten,* Zweiter Theil (Hamm, 1830), as indicated in the text, but Ernest E. Austen's *A Monograph of the Tsetse-Flies* (London: British Museum (Natural History), 1903; New York: Johnson Reprint, 1966) affords the best starting point for investigating the ramifications of early taxonomic studies on these flies.

Pages 13–19

Two books by Claude Fuller were central to an examination of the first confrontations of European newcomers with tsetse in South Africa—*Tsetse in the Transvaal and Surrounding Territories: An Historical Review* (Pretoria: Government Printing and Stationery Office, 1923; Entomology Memoirs, No. 1) and *Louis Trigardt's Trek across the Drakensberg, 1837–1838,* edited by Leo Fouche (Cape Town: Van Riebeeck Society, 1932). For general background on the area and the times I also made use of two books by Eric A. Walker—*A History of Southern Africa,* 3d ed., reissued with corrections (London, New York: Longmans, 1959) and the more specific *The Great Trek* (London: A. and C. Black, 1934). Although I have focused here on the Voortrekkers and the ivory hunters, the search for gold was also important in the area during this period—and the prospectors also encountered tsetse, as Fuller details in the first of his two books mentioned above.

I have quoted from page viii of his Introduction in Volume I and from pages 182 and 227 of Volume II of an edition of Roualeyn Gordon Cumming's *Five Years of a Hunter's Life in the Far Interior of South Africa . . . ,* 2 vols. (New York: Harper, 1871; originally published, 1850), and from "The Elephant's Child" in Rudyard Kipling's immortal *Just So Stories* (New York: Doubleday, Doran, 1902), p. 67. Charles E. Carrington's *The Life of Rudyard Kipling* (Garden City, N.Y.: Doubleday, 1955) tells of Kipling's experiences in Africa.

I tried to pin tsetse and its trypanosomes to the well-known fever tree as responsible for giving that tall, graceful acacia with its smooth greenish-yellow bark its unfortunate name, but the evidence did not accrue. Too many fevers—among them, malaria—have their origin among the mosquitoes and flies that frequent the river courses and the moist lowlands where this tree thrives. Actually, ambiguity exists about the meaning of the name fever tree; some think it means to ward off, others to bring on, fever.

Isaac Schapera's *The Tswana* (London: International African Institute, 1953; Ethnographic Survey of Africa: Southern Africa, Part III) is the standard work about these peoples. Two books written in popular vein about African leaders mentioned in this section express a European viewpoint—Peter Becker's *Path of Blood: The Rise and Conquests of Mzilikazi, Founder of the Matabele Tribe of Southern Africa* (London: Longmans, 1962) and Anthony Sillery's *Sechele: The Story of an African Chief* (Oxford: George Ronald, 1954).

William Cotton Oswell, Hunter and Explorer: The Story of His Life with Certain Correspondence and Extracts from the Private Journal of David Livingstone, Hitherto Unpublished (London: William Heinemann, 1900) is W. Edward Oswell's two-volume biography of his father. I have quoted from pages 135–138 of this work. Oswell and such other well-known hunters as Frederick J. Jackson —of later East Africa fame—and Frederick Courteney Selous contributed pieces to the second edition of Clive Phillipps-Wolley's two-volume *Big Game Shooting* (London: Longmans, Green, 1901). Those who are interested in reading more about ivory may refer to George Frederick Kunz, *Ivory and the Elephant in Art, in Archaeology, and in Science* (Garden City, N.Y.: Doubleday, Page, 1916), and to R. W. Beachey, "The East African ivory trade in the nineteenth century," *Journal of African History* 8 (2): 269–290, 1967. In the *Encyclopaedia Britannica* (1949) article on "Plastics" Charles A. Breskin describes how decimation of elephant herds in India and in Africa in the nineteenth century to supply ivory for billiard balls and piano keys stimulated chemists in the United States and elsewhere to invent celluloid and to build a plastics industry that today provides countless substitutes for ivory.

In Austen's *Monograph* . . . (1903, 1966), one finds reference to Vardon's role in identifying tsetse. John O. Westwood quoted Vardon's statement regarding the specimens Vardon gave him (page

141) and described *G. morsitans* in "Observations on the destructive species of Dipterous Insects known in Africa under the names of the Tsetse, Zimb, and Tsaltsalya, and on their supposed connexion with the Fourth Plague of Egypt" *Annals and Magazine of Natural History*, ser. 2, Vol. 10, no. LVI: 138–150, 1852, also published in *Proceedings of the Zoological Society of London*, Part XVIII: 258–270, 1850.

Pages 19–29

Roland Oliver's *The Missionary Factor in East Africa* (London and New York: Longmans, Green, 1952) is an excellent source for missionary philosophies and the missionary impact in East Africa. The state of medical knowledge in Livingstone's time and its influence on British penetration of Africa may be found in Philip Curtin's important study, *The Image of Africa* (Madison: University of Wisconsin Press, 1964).

Livingstone, the Doctor: His Life and Travels (Oxford: Basil Blackwell, 1957) by the prolific doctor-writer Michael Gelfand proved to be especially valuable in the preparation of the material on Livingstone; there is also an unsigned article entitled "Livingstone's contributions to medicine," *Nature* 208 (5015): 1050–1051, December 11, 1965, based on an article by Gelfand published earlier in 1965. Livingstone's comments on the relationship between geographical exploration and missionary enterprise and the importance to him of finding the sources of the Nile come from pages 378 and 381 of John Butt, "David Livingstone and the idea of African evolution," *History Today* 12 (6): 376–382, June 1963.

David Livingstone's famous book, *Missionary Travels and Researches in South Africa* (London: John Murray, 1857; New York: Harper, 1858), still eminently readable, is the source of his description of the tsetse's bite as well as much else about Livingstone; on page 96 (1858 ed.) Livingstone speculated that a bulb at the root of the tsetse's proboscis contained a poison-germ. During the 1860's, Livingstone was also searching for a route to the interior that was outside Portuguese territory; he found this in the Rovuma (Ruvuma) River, now the border between Tanzania and Mozambique, which he explored in several trips during that decade. George Shepperson has edited Livingstone's diaries of these trips and provided much explanatory material in *David Livingstone and the Rovuma* (Edinburgh: University Press, 1965). The first work undertaken by Livingstone after his resignation from the London Missionary Society was the expedition to the Zambezi, a British-government-sponsored effort to open up a way to the interior of that part of Africa with a view to possible future white settlement. Some of the important questions in the minds of the government —and the explorers—concerned tsetse and whether it would prove a barrier to such settlement. These matters, and the use of quinine as both prophylactic and cure in man's fight against malaria, are treated in David and Charles Livingstone's *Narrative of an Expedition to the Zambesi and Its Tributaries; and of the Discovery of the Lakes Shirwa and Nyassa, 1858–1864* (London: John Murray, 1865; New York: Harper, 1866), and in *The Zambesi Doctors: David Livingstone's Letters to John Kirk, 1858–1872* (Edinburgh: University Press, 1964), edited by R. Foskett. On page 368 (1865 ed.) and page 389 (1866 ed.) of *Narrative of an Expedition to the Zambesi . . .* Livingstone noted that "myriads of musquitoes showed" malaria's presence.

Pages 29–35

A number of Henry Stanley's writings are indispensable to the story of the spread of sleeping sickness from Stanley Pool up the Congo River. *How I Found Livingstone: Travels, Adventures and Discoveries in Central Africa: including an Account of Four Months' Residence with Dr. Livingstone* (New York: Scribner, Armstrong, 1873), on page 412 of which we find "Dr. Livingstone, I presume?," is one of these. Page 91 contains his description of the damage done to animals by "chufwa." Stanley's job description for the sort of missionary who would be of service in Uganda comes from his book *Through the Dark Continent, or The Sources of the Nile . . .* (New York: Harper, 1878), I, 209. H. B. Thomas speculates upon Stanley's letter suggesting Buganda as a mission field in "Ernest Linant de Bellefonds and Stanley's letter to the

'Daily Telegraph,' " *Uganda Journal* 2 (1): 7–13, July 1934. *The Congo, and the Founding of Its Free State,* 2 vols. (New York: Harper, 1885), by Stanley is an additional useful source, among others.

Years before Stanley explored the Congo, Thomas M. Winterbottom had written about sleeping sickness in his two-volume *An Account of the Native Africans in the Neighbourhood of Sierra Leone; to Which Is Added, an Account of the Present State of Medicine among Them* (London, 1803); I have quoted from page 29 of Volume II of this work. Like Adam Afzelius, who collected the type specimen of tsetse, Winterbottom was in the employ of the Sierra Leone Company in the last decade of the eighteenth century. Unlike John Atkins, Winterbottom made a real—if not always successful—effort to understand Africans; his work deserves a wider audience.

The earliest monograph on sleeping sickness known to me is a thesis which Paul-Marie-Auguste Guérin, a French naval doctor in the West Indies, submitted for the doctorate of the Faculty of Medicine, Paris, in 1869. In *De la maladie du sommeil* (Paris: A. Parent, 1869; Faculté de Médecine de Paris, No. 201), Guérin hypothesized that sleeping sickness might have originated in the Congo, since so many of the slaves he had treated for it had told him they came from there. In 1876–1877, at official government request, another French medical man, Armand Corré, undertook investigations of the disease in Senegal; the curious may be interested in his "Contribution a l'étude de la maladie du sommeil (hypnose)," *Gazette Medicale de Paris,* No. 46: 545–547, 11 Novembre, 1876, and "Recherches sur la maladie du sommeil," *Archives de médecine navale* 27: 292–312 and 330–356, 1877, and in "Journal du docteur Corré en pays sérère (décembre 1876–janvier 1877)" edited by G. Debien, in *Bulletin de l'Institut Français d'Afrique Noire* ser. B, 26 (3–4): 532–600, 1964. By that time Albert A. Gore had published "The sleeping sickness of western Africa" in the *British Medical Journal,* Jan. 2, 1875: 5–7. Soon afterward, sleeping sickness had found its way into at least one important medical textbook, August Hirsch's three-volume *Handbook of Geo-*

graphical and Historical Pathology, translated by Charles Creighton (London, 1883–1886), III: 595–602.

Tippu Tib—there are various spellings—was one of the most influential black men in nineteenth-century Africa, and he turns up in many history books. A German doctor, Heinrich Brode, prepared *Tippoo Tib: The Story of His Career in Central Africa,* translated by H. Havelock (London: Edward Arnold, 1907), from Tippu's own accounts. More recently Tippu's recollections in Swahili, *Maisha ya Hamed bin Muhammed el Murjebi yaani Tippu Tip,* translated by W. H. Whiteley, were published as a supplement to the *East African Swahili Committee Journal* 28, 29, July 1958 and January 1959. A passage from these recollections entitled "The Arrival of Stanley" can be found in *A Selection of African Prose: I, Traditional Oral Texts,* compiled by Whiteley (Oxford: Clarendon Press, 1964), pp. 107–112.

Vachel Lindsay, who, like Edgar Rice Burroughs of Tarzan fame, never set foot on African soil, certainly must have done his homework well to depict as he did the Congo River and its people in his poem "The Congo," from *Collected Poems of Vachel Lindsay* (Copyright 1914 by The Macmillan Company, renewed 1942 by Elizabeth C. Lindsay). Although "The Congo," based on Lindsay's familiarity with the southern part of the Mississippi River, displays an attitude toward the Negro race not in tune with modern thinking, the poem is well worth reading for certain intuitive impressions Lindsay has recorded that do in fact seem relevant to the Congo River, which may seem a giant muddy trough when viewed from its banks, or a shredded ribbon when seen from the air through the haze of burning tropical jungle, but always a river "CUTTING THROUGH THE FOREST WITH A GOLDEN TRACK" (pages 3–4) to those who love it.

Pages 35–37

E. J. Glave's *Six Years of Adventure in Congo-Land* (London: Sampson Low, Marston, 1893), provides a vivid if optimistic picture of conditions in the area during the period which concerns us here. Material quoted is from pages 140 and 141.

Pages 37–43

The correspondence between Roger Casement and Manson is noted in Philip H. Manson-Bahr and A. Alcock, *The Life and Work of Sir Patrick Manson* (London, Cassell, 1927); Casement's description of the local treatment for sleeping sickness has been quoted from page 111. The portion of Casement's famous report which included the statements of the missionary Whitehead and other descriptions of sleeping sickness (material quoted will be found on pages 21, 23, 64, and 65) was published by the British Foreign Office under the title *Correspondence and Report from His Majesty's Consul at Boma Respecting the Administration of the Independent State of the Congo* (London, H.M.S.O., 1904; Africa No. 1 (1904), Cd. 1933); the two later sections are not of interest for our purpose. Casement's comments about the Sanford mission and Joseph Conrad's assessment of Casement are from pages 36 and 29 respectively of Denis Gwynn, *Traitor or Patriot: The Life and Death of Roger Casement* (New York: Jonathan Cape and Harrison Smith, 1931).

William Roger Louis explored what he called Casement's "apocalyptic vision of evil in the Congo" in "Roger Casement and the Congo," *Journal of African History* 5 (1): 99–120, 1964. There is also an article by James P. White on "The Sanford Exploring Expedition," *Journal of African History* 8 (2): 291–302, 1967.

The Dutton-Todd-Christy efforts in the Congo are well documented: J. Everett Dutton, John L. Todd, and Cuthbert Christy, *Reports of the Trypanosomiasis Expedition to the Congo, 1903–1904 . . .* (London: Williams and Norgate for the University Press of Liverpool, 1904; Liverpool School of Tropical Medicine —Memoir XIII). There is also an article by Michel F. Lechat, "L'expédition Dutton-Todd au Congo (1903–1905)—de Boma à Coquilhatville (septembre 1903–juillet 1904)," *Annales de la Société belge de Médecine tropicale* 44 (3): 493–511, 1964, which is based on material from the Todd archives.

The quotation from Joseph Conrad's novella *Heart of Darkness*, originally published early this century, can be found on page 82 (New York: New American Library, 1950).

Pages 43–54

It is a pity that so colorful a character as R. S. S. Baden-Powell, alias B-P of *"Be Prepared"* fame of the Boy Scout movement, for reasons of relevance cannot occupy a central role in our story of the stresses and strains rinderpest, nagana, and tsetse flies set up in competing among themselves for the animal population of greater eastern Africa. Baden-Powell's comments about the jigger have been quoted from page 448 of his *The Matabele Campaign, 1896, Being a Narrative of the Campaign in Suppressing the Native Rising in Matabeleland and Mashonaland* (London: Methuen, 1897). E. E. Reynolds wrote *Baden-Powell: A Biography of Lord Baden-Powell of Gilwell* (London: Oxford University Press, 1943). The famous hunter Frederick C. Selous—like Baden-Powell—described the rinderpest in his account of the Matabele Campaign, *Sunshine and Storm in Rhodesia* (London: Rowe and Ward, 1896).

R. W. M. Mettam, in "A short history of rinderpest with special reference to Africa," *Uganda Journal* 5 (1): 22–26, July 1937, and Ford and Hall quote Lugard, page 23 of Mettam's article being the source of his statement regarding the tremendous number of cattle deaths. Margery Perham, his biographer, has edited *The Diaries of Lord Lugard*, of which volumes I–III (Evanston: Northwestern University Press, 1959) cover his experiences in East Africa from 1889 to 1892.

H. F. Morris' *The Heroic Recitations of the Bahima of Ankole* (Oxford: Clarendon Press, 1964) contains a helpful historical review of the depredations of rinderpest, smallpox, and tsetse in that part of Uganda, as well as a praise poem composed in a later time of disease and drought (about 1918).

For the East African rinderpest outbreak of the 1890's, I relied heavily on "The History of Karagwe (Bukoba District)," by John Ford and R. de Z. Hall, *Tanganyika Notes and Records*, No. 24: 3–27, 1947. "Tripping down the greensward" is quoted from page 23 of this article, Stuhlman's comment about the Bahima having to engage in agriculture and Lugard's description of those who survived rinderpest are from page 20, and Baumann's observations on the Masai are from page 21. Such histories are an increasing, and welcome, trend in African historiography. Another one which was useful with respect to Emin Pasha and the areas treated is A. R. Dunbar, *A History of Bunyoro-Kitara* (Nairobi: Oxford University Press for the East African Institute of Social Research, 1965).

Emin Pasha is my favorite European in the Africa of colonial days because of the mysterious aura that enshrouds this complex man, an aura that probably never will be completely dispersed. Georg Schweitzer's *Emin Pasha, His Life and Work, Compiled from His Journals, Letters, Scientific Notes, and from Official Documents*, 2 vols. (London, 1898; reprinted New York: Negro Universities Press, 1969), is interesting enough as a chronicle of his life and work, but it does not do justice to the drama of Emin Pasha's life. Schweitzer registers Emin Pasha's complaint about being a rolling stone on page 230 of his second volume. This query, coupled with the rinderpest outbreak, identifies another theme which I have pursued in the text—that of man aiding and abetting perforce the diseases which are his own worst enemies. Those interested in Emin may also consult *Emin Pasha in Central Africa, Being a Collection of His Letters and Journals* edited by G. Schweinfurth and others, and translated by Mrs. Robert W. Felkin (London: George Philip and Son, 1888).

H. M. Stanley's two-volume *Through the Dark Continent* (1878) also deals with the period and area in question. His *In Darkest Africa, or The Quest, Rescue, and Retreat of Emin, Governor of Equatoria* (London: Samuel Low, Marston, 1890 and 1897) of famous title is specifically concerned with the Emin Pasha Relief Expedition, as is Olivia Manning's *The Reluctant Rescue* (Garden City, N.Y.: Doubleday, 1947), a popularized account published by Heinemann the same year in England as *Remarkable Expedition*.

At least two other accounts of the expedition (both firsthand) may also be commended: *The Diary of A. J. Mounteney Jephson: Emin Pasha Relief Expedition, 1887–1889*, edited by Dorothy Middleton (Cambridge, Cambridge University Press for the Hakluyt Society, 1969), and Thomas Heazle Parke, *My Personal Experiences in Equatorial Africa as Medical Officer of the Emin Pasha Relief Expedition* (New York: Charles Scribner, 1891). Parke does not discuss either sleeping sickness or tsetse in his book, but his accounts of the deaths of some of the party are suggestive.

Alan Moorehead's *The White Nile* (New York: Harper, 1960) provides highly readable accounts of the expedition, the early explorers, and the entire setting. His *The Blue Nile* (New York: Harper and Row, 1962) is also warmly recommended, although it is not as germane to this chapter as the earlier work.

Richard F. Burton described his experiences in the area in the two-volume *The Lake Regions of Central Africa* (London, 1860), which has recently been republished (New York: Horizon Press, 1961).

Pages 54–55

On animal disease in general, I found the most helpful single source to be Michiel Wilhelm Henning's *Animal Diseases in South Africa*, 3d ed. (Johannesburg, Central News Agency, 1956). Fuller's *Tsetse in the Transvaal . . .* (1923) was also important. Others include J. Carmichael, "The virus of rinderpest and its relation to *Glossina morsitans*, Westw.," *Bulletin of Entomological Research* 24: 337–342, September 1933; P. J. du Toit, "Game in relation to animal diseases," *Journal of the South African Veterinary Medical Association* 18: 59–66, 1947; H. E. Hornby, "The control of animal diseases in relation to overstocking and soil erosion," *Empire Journal of Experimental Agriculture* 5 (18): 143–153, 1937; and a two-part article in the same volume of the same journal: J. Smith, "The combating of animal diseases and the improvement of stock in Empire countries," *ibid.*, Nos. 17 and 18: 19–28 and 133–142, 1937.

W. E. F. Thomson, "Historical fragments on trypanosomiasis and the spread of sleeping-sickness to British East Africa," *East African Medical Journal* 37 (11): 724–730, November 1960, and the 1961 "Correspondence" about it, *ibid.* 38 (1): 55–56; (2): 90–92; (5): 266–267; (9): 432–434; and (10): 466, deal with the question of whether sleeping sickness had existed in East Africa prior to Stanley's arrival on the Emin Pasha Relief Expedition, among other matters.

Pages 55–58

Winston Churchill's description of the lakeshore region of Uganda I have quoted from page 103 of *My African Journey* (New York and London: Hodder and Stoughton, 1908). Other "Churchillian" assessments of Uganda are equally vivid and germane to our story. After he witnessed the ravages of the sleeping sickness epidemic in the area around Lake Victoria, he termed Uganda a "beautiful garden of death," according to Mona Macmillan's *Introducing East Africa*, 2d ed. (London: Faber and Faber, 1955), p. 37. Uganda and Ugandans survived the epidemic. They also withstood much political and religious strife in the decades before and after the sleeping sickness epidemic. Today Kampala, the capital of Uganda, seemingly sleepy a year or two ago, sustains political stress centered on one of its seven hills where parliament is situated. At the same time it supports an elite university with lofty ideals on another. Still, Kampala with its benign climate, lush vegetation, and flowers epitomizes the Uganda people like to liken to a garden.

Many different authors have described the sleeping sickness epidemic of the late 1890's around Lake Victoria. Material about and by the Cooks, especially Sir Albert, has been most useful. Sir Albert was the author of a book entitled *Uganda Memories (1897–1940)* (Kampala: Uganda Society, 1945) as well as "The journey to Uganda in 1896 and Kampala during the closing years of the last century," *Uganda Journal* 1 (2): 83–95, April 1934, and "Further memories of Uganda," *ibid.* 2 (2): 97–115, October 1934; "How sleeping sickness came to Uganda," *East African Medical Journal* 17 (10): 408–413, January 1941; and "The medical history of Uganda," *ibid.* 13 (3): 66–81, June 1936, and 13 (4): 99–110, July 1936.

CHAPTER II—ASKING THE RIGHT QUESTIONS

The period from 1890 to World War I encompassed a knowledge explosion in tropical medicine and related fields; the findings of Bruce are by no means the only examples. The reader can review the state of science circa 1900 in reference books of the period—for example, the articles on "Entomology" written by George H. Carpenter, "Medicine" by Sir Thomas C. Allbutt, and "Science" by William C. Whetham in the *Encyclopaedia Britannica*, 11th ed. (1911). For entomology, the histories by E. O. Essig (1931) and L. O. Howard (1930) have already been suggested; for tropical medicine, I have found three articles particularly useful: George Carmichael Low, "A retrospect of tropical medicine from 1894 to 1914," *Transactions of the Royal Society of Tropical Medicine and Hygiene* 23 (3): 213–234, November 25, 1929; Philip Manson-Bahr, "The march of tropical medicine during the last fifty years (Footprints on the sands of time)," *ibid.* 52 (6): 483–499, November 28, 1958; and M. A. Soltys, "Golden jubilee of the discovery of sleeping sickness in East Africa," *East African Medical Journal* 30 (9): 389–392, September 1953.

Also worthy of note are another article by Low, "The history of the foundation of the Society of Tropical Medicine and Hygiene," *Transactions of the Royal Society of Tropical Medicine and Hygiene* 22 (2): 197–202, August 1928; Raymond E. Dumett, "The campaign against malaria and the expansion of scientific medical and sanitary services in British West Africa, 1898–1910," *African Historical Studies* 1 (2): 153–197, 1968; and R. L. Sheppard, "Tropical Diseases Bulletin, Volume Fifty," *Tropical Diseases Bulletin* 50 (1): 1–2, January 1953. Ann Beck wrote a book-length monograph entitled *A History of the British Medical Administration of East Africa, 1900–1950* (Cambridge: Harvard University Press, 1970).

The London and the Liverpool schools of tropical medicine founded within months of each other in 1898 have been the subjects of books, notably the Liverpool School of Tropical Medicine, *Historical Record, 1898–1920* (Liverpool: Liverpool University Press, 1920) and Philip Manson-Bahr, *History of the School of Tropical Medicine in London (1899–1949)* (London: H. K. Lewis, 1956; London School of Hygiene and Tropical Medicine, Memoir No. 11). How these two schools vied with each other for field assignments for their staff and for government and other financing at home makes fascinating reading.

Preliminary Report

ON THE

TSETSE FLY DISEASE OR NAGANA,

IN ZULULAND.

BY

SURGEON-MAJOR DAVID BRUCE, A.M.S.

Ubombo, Zululand,
December, 1895.

Bennett & Davis, Printers, Field Street, Durban.

Facsimile of title page and letter of transmittal, David Bruce's preliminary report to Sir Walter Hely-Hutchinson.

To His Excellency

The Hon. Sir Walter Hely-Hutchinson, K.C.M.G.,

Governor of Natal and Zululand, &c., &c.

Your Excellency,—I have the honour to inform you that in accordance with instructions received from you, I left Pietermaritzburg on the 21st August, 1895, and arrived at Ubombo, Zululand, on the 8th September, 1895, for the purpose of continuing the investigation of the Tsetse Fly Disease, or Nagana, as it occurs in Zululand.

I have now the honour to forward a Preliminary Report, containing a statement of the results of the investigation up to the present date.

I may here state that on my arrival in Zululand the Tsetse Fly Disease and Nagana were looked upon as separate and distinct diseases, and one of the first results of this investigation was to show that they are undoubtedly one and the same.

This Preliminary Report contains :—

1.—A description of the Hæmatozoon discovered by me in 1894, in the blood of animals affected by this disease, a parasite not previously discovered in Africa.

2.—A description of the Tsetse Fly, with experiments designed to show the part (if any) this Fly takes in the causation of the disease.

3.—The result of experiments having for their object, proof of the connection (if any) which is supposed to exist between the Big Game and the spread of the disease.

4.—A description of the disease as it affects domestic animals, with illustrative cases.

5.—Inoculation and feeding experiments to show the communicability of the disease from affected to healthy animals.

I have the honour to be,
Sir,
Your most obedient Servant,
DAVID BRUCE,
Surgeon-Major A.M.S.

Ubombo,
Zululand, 12th December, 1895.

Pages 59–68

The early part of Chapter II concentrates on Bruce's work. The quotation at the beginning, found on page 2 of Bruce's *Preliminary Report on the Tsetse Fly Disease, or Nagana, in Zululand* (Durban: Bennett and Davis, 1895), is intended to illustrate that a certain amount of doctrinaire speculation is an essential ingredient to the right mix of preconceived notions and methodology in order to achieve results in science as in any other discipline. This theme pervades the chapter; this mix works sometimes toward obtaining valid results, and sometimes not.

Written in 1895, Bruce's preliminary report exhibits certain old-fashioned frills in presentation and in format which make it interesting to compare with modern documents on scientific matters presented to the public. These matters of style were the order of the day in Bruce's time but I like to pretend that the respect with which Bruce addresses Sir Walter Hely-Hutchinson has a deeper significance in showing pride for the superb work he had accomplished and that by displaying so many different styles of type on the title page the local printer in Durban not only advertises what his printing shop can do but also may be responding to a premonition that the report itself would become, as it did, a classic in the development of the science of parasitology. This report has served as my main source for information about Bruce and his methods; passages quoted, in the order of their appearance in the text, have been taken from pages 6, 28, 8, 7, and 8.

Bruce's *Further Report on the Tsetse Fly Disease or Nagana, in Zululand* (London: Harrison and Sons, 1896) was helpful. Two articles were especially important: William MacArthur's "An account of some of Sir David Bruce's researches, based on his own manuscript notes," *Transactions of the Royal Society of Tropical Medicine and Hygiene* 49 (5): 404–412, September 30, 1955, and Muriel Robertson's "Some aspects of trypanosomiasis with particular reference to the work of Sir David Bruce," *Journal of Tropical Medicine and Hygiene* 59 (4): 69–77, April 1956. I have also made use of the biographical sketch in Volume II of the 1942 edition of

H. Harold Scott's *History of Tropical Medicine* and the obituary of Bruce by A. E. Hamerton in *Transactions of the Royal Society of Tropical Medicine and Hygiene* 25: 305–312, January 1932. E. E. Austen's *A Monograph of the Tsetse-Flies* (1966) provided two quotations: the description of *G. pallidipes*, page 88, and the collector's note, page 89.

The reports and documents that Miss Widenmann examined in the Public Record Office, London, and the Bruce papers that were kindly made available to us at the Royal Society of Tropical Medicine and Hygiene were of interest, though they did not produce additional details relevant to Bruce's assignment in Zululand.

The history of the railroads has been chronicled by Mervyn F. Hill in a two-part work bearing the overall title of *Permanent Way*. Volume I is *The Story of the Kenya and Uganda Railway* and Volume II *The Story of the Tanganyika Railways*, both published in Nairobi by East African Railways and Harbours, the first in 1950 and the second in 1960.

Pages 68–75

J. N. P. Davies, when he was in the Department of Pathology of the Medical School of Makerere College (now Makerere University), wrote a provocative two-part article "The cause of sleeping-sickness?," *East African Medical Journal* 39 (3): 81–99, March 1962, and 39 (4): 145–160, April 1962. Davies made a strong case for the field men of the 1900's who were trying to elucidate the cause of sleeping sickness during the Uganda epidemic and who might have done more, given time and opportunity, than the men in London who pontificated about the cause of sleeping sickness and formed commissions of experts to look into the problem. He may have gone too far in this direction, but his articles nevertheless are a mainstay for the study of the cause of sleeping sickness as I have told it. More recently, Harvey G. Soff has conducted an historical inquiry into the epidemic in general and has published an article entitled "Sleeping sickness in the Lake Victoria region of British East Africa, 1900–1915," *African Historical Studies* 2 (2): 255–268, 1969. Reference may also be made again to the article by

W. E. F. Thomson entitled "Historical fragments on trypanosomiasis and the spread of sleeping-sickness to British East Africa"
(1960).

Sir Albert has been the subject of two book-length biographies,
Joyce Reason's *Safety Last* (London: Highway Press, 1954) and the
less-popularized *That Good Physician,* by Brian O'Brien (London:
Hodder and Stoughton, 1962). The biographical note by W. R. Bil-
lington and "Appreciations" by other former colleagues published
shortly after Sir Albert's death in *East African Medical Journal* 28
(10): 397–401 and 423–427, October 1951, are of particular interest.

The phrase about "the divining-rod of a preconceived idea" is
from page 130 of Philip H. Manson-Bahr and A. Alcock's *Life and
Work of Sir Patrick Manson* (1927), which I have used as the chief
source on Sir Patrick Manson. There are also the address "The
Manson Saga" by Manson-Bahr and a series of other centennial
tributes all published in *Transactions of the Royal Society of Tropical Medicine and Hygiene* 38 (6): 401–424, July 1945. Manson's
famous textbook is *Tropical Diseases: A Manual of the Diseases of
Warm Climates* (New York: William Wood, 1898). The early London sleeping sickness cases and Sir Patrick's connection with them
—among many other points—were discussed by F. M. Sandwith in
three numbers of *Medical Press* for 1912: "Cattle trypanosomiasis
and the early history of sleeping sickness" (April 3: 349–353), "The
later history of sleeping sickness" (April 10: 374–379), and "What
we know to-day about sleeping sickness" (April 17: 402–407). The
first sleeping sickness case thoroughly studied in London—by Manson and others—was described by the principal physician on the
case, Stephen Mackenzie, in "On a case of 'Negro Lethargy' or 'the
sleeping sickness' of Africa," Clinical Society of London, *Transactions,* 24: 41–57, 1890–91. Soon after his association with this patient and another treated by Mackenzie, Manson published his *Filaria* theory of sleeping sickness in "The geographical distribution,
pathological relations, and life history of filaria sanguinis hominis
diurna and of filaria sanguinis hominis perstans, in connexion with
preventive medicine," International Congress of Hygiene and De-

mography, *Transactions*, 1891: 79–97. He repeated the theory in contributions on sleeping sickness to at least two textbooks prior to the publication of his own manual: *A System of Medicine, by Many Writers*, 9 vols., edited by Thomas Clifford Allbutt (New York and London: Macmillan, 1897) II, 479–486; and Andrew Davidson, ed., *Hygiene and Diseases of Warm Climates* (Edinburgh and London: Young J. Pentland, 1893), 503–510.

"Dr. Jack's" famous article announcing the first cases in the Uganda epidemic was J. Howard Cook, "Notes on cases of 'sleeping sickness' occurring in the Uganda Protectorate," *Journal of Tropical Medicine*, July 15, 1901: 236–239.

The material in the text about selecting members to form a scientific commission comes from a variety of sources but, in the main, from the J. N. P. Davies articles. This material points toward a fundamental axiom—there is no such thing as an objective commission organized to study a scientific problem. In Manson's as well as in our own time, the outcome of the deliberations of any commission is preordained by the choice of the commission members and their frame of reference.

Aldo Castellani wrote a breezy autobiography entitled *A Doctor in Many Lands* (Garden City, N.Y.: Doubleday, 1960). He related the story of his purchase of his tropical outfit, including the sun hat, on page 36. The passage that deals with his selection of clothing prompts one to consider broadly man's instinct to protect himself from insects through the use of clothes mainly but also of cosmetics. There may be original and residual motivations that influence the style and kind of clothes and cosmetics one uses. We know garments are used in other parts of the world sometimes for protection against insect attack as well as against the harshness of the environment. It seems logical to me at least to infer that the use of mascara in the form of antimony, a poison, about the eyes of those who live in the dry areas of Africa and in the Middle East may have originated as a protection against face flies. The men in Masailand who construct coiffures that resemble mud palaces on their heads at one time may have treated their hair with mud (ocher) to keep insects away. Except in certain isolated and specific instances fully described in the text, however, efforts to associate the use of clothes and of cosmetics as protective devices for tsetse fly bites have been nonproductive.

C. A. Wiggins' "Early days in British East Africa and Uganda" appeared in *East African Medical Journal* 37 (11): 699–708, November 1960, and (12): 780–793, December 1960); his comments about the first commission are quoted from page 704.

Pages 75–84

The sources already cited that relate to Castellani, Bruce, Manson, and Davies are the basis for the continuation of the story of the activities of the second sleeping sickness commission. Castellani's discovery of the "fish-like parasite" is recounted on page 60 of his *A Doctor in Many Lands* (1960). The characterization of Nabarro as "rather mild and retiring" comes from page 98 of the first part of J. N. P. Davies' article, "The cause of sleeping-sickness?" (1962).

In addition, one should refer to Julien Brault, who published his speculation about the relationship between trypanosomes and sleeping sickness (and tsetse flies) in a footnote to his "Contribution à la géographie médicale des maladies africaines," *Janus: Archives internationales pour l'histoire de la médecine et la géographie médicale* 3: 36–42, 1898. Sir Hesketh Bell's comments about Ray Lankester are quoted from page 98 of his *Glimpses of a Governor's Life from Diaries, Letters and Memoranda* (London: Sampson Low, Marston, 1946).

Both volumes of the *British Medical Journal* for 1903 contain numerous articles on the sleeping sickness epidemic and speculations about the cause of the disease. Of particular interest are "Etiology of sleeping sickness" (Vol. I: 617–618, March 14, 1903) from the latter page of which Castellani's announcement that he considered his special bacterium the cause has been excerpted; "Trypanosomiasis and its cause" (Vol. I: 721–722, March 28, 1903) in which Alexander Maxwell-Adams, Jr., suggested the relationship between trypanosomiasis—which he thought might be transmitted by a flea—and sleeping sickness; C. J. Baker's "Three cases of trypanosoma in man in Entebbe, Uganda" (Vol. I: 1254–1256, May 30, 1903), the final page of which is the source of the quotation about Bruce's assuring Baker his fly was of the tsetse group; and "The etiology of sleeping sickness" (Vol. II: 1343–1350, Nov. 21, 1903), which reports rather fully the observations and conclusions Bruce, Nabarro, and Captain Greig made in their *Further Report on Sleeping Sickness in Uganda.* Bruce's statement that the evidence indicated "trypanosoma fever the first stage of sleeping sickness" comes from page 1345, his conclusions ending with "sleeping sickness is, in short, a human tsetse-fly disease" from page 1344 of this article. J. N. P. Davies reported the German note on *Trypanosome castellanii* on page 153 of the second part of his article, "The cause of sleeping-sickness?" (1962).

Pages 84–99

After the cause of sleeping sickness became known, a number of loose ends remained to be tied. Sir Albert Cook's descriptions of the treatments he used for sleeping sickness have been quoted from page 163 of his *Uganda Memories* (Kampala: Uganda Society, 1945). Robert Koch and his efforts to develop a control measure for sleeping sickness figure into this stage of development. I think it is especially noteworthy that at sixty-four, close to the end of his career, he was prepared to "rough it" on an island in Lake Victoria in order to conduct research on sleeping sickness. The information about the work of Robert Koch comes chiefly from three sources: M. E. M. Walker's *Pioneers of Public Health* (New York: Macmillan, 1930); an obituary by "C. J. M." in the Smithsonian Institution's *Annual Report of the Board of Regents, 1911* (Washington, D.C.: GPO, 1912), pp. 651–658, reprinted from *Proceedings of the Royal Society, London,* ser. B, 83 (B567): xviii–xxiv, May 31, 1911; and *The Baganda at Home,* written by a prominent CMS missionary of the period, Charles W. Hattersley (London: Religious Tract Society, 1908; reprint New York: Barnes and Noble, 1968; London: Frank Cass, 1968).

More on arsenic and on atoxyl will be found in Chapter III. In drawing upon Austen's *A Monograph of the Tsetse-Flies* (1966), I have quoted from pages 3 and 4 to describe distinguishing features of different species of tsetse. Bernhard and Michael Grzimek on pages 292 and 295 of their book *Serengeti Shall Not Die* (New York: E. P. Dutton, 1961) give about as vivid a description of the life cycle of the tsetse flies as one can find anywhere. The description of *G. palpalis* and its habitat comes mainly from C. B. Symes, "Outline of work on *G. palpalis* in Kenya," *East African Medical Journal* 12 (9): 263–281, December 1935.

According to T. D. A. Cockerell's "New species of North American fossil beetles, cockroaches, and tsetse flies" in the *Proceedings of the United States National Museum* 54 (2337): 301–311, 1919, George N. Rohwer found a fossil fly in the shale beds at Florissant, Colorado, in 1907. Cockerell identified it as a tsetse fly. E. E. Austen verified Cockerell's identification from descriptions and drawings of this fly. Cockerell described a second specimen of tsetse found in these beds and named it *Glossina osborni*. Two additional specimens were found in 1916 in the same beds by George Wilson.

"Venezuela arms against Chagas' disease" on pages 26 (the source of the quote about *R. prolixus*) and 27 of *World Health* for November 1969 characterizes Chagas' disease as a national problem in Venezuela and describes the life cycle of the insect *Rhodnius prolixus* that transmits it. For a more thorough treatment of trypanosomiasis in Africa and the Americas, the student of parasitology ought to consult WHO's Technical Report No. 411, *Comparative Studies of American and African Trypanosomiasis* (Geneva: World Health Organization, 1969).

Leonard Engel discusses Charles Darwin's possible illness from Chagas' disease in his introduction and annotations to Darwin's *The Voyage of the Beagle* (Garden City, N.Y.: Doubleday Anchor Books, 1962)—a theory put forward in 1959 by Dr. S. Adler of the Hebrew University of Jerusalem.

F. K. Kleine, a German scientist working in Tanganyika, first recognized the significance of the time it took for trypanosomes to pass through the fly and correlated this integral relationship with their vector with the infectivity of trypanosomes to man. (See F. K. Kleine, "Positive Infektionsversuche mit Trypanosoma brucei durch Glossina palpalis," *Deutsche Medizinische Wochenschrift* 35 (11): 469–470, March 18, 1909.) Subsequently Muriel Robertson, A. E. Hamerton and Bruce, among others, elucidated this relationship. Lorande L. Woodruff's article "Protozoa" in the 1949 edition of the *Encyclopaedia Britannica* contains a diagram of the life cycle of *T. gambiense* (18: 630).

CHAPTER III—CAMPAIGNS AGAINST TSETSE AND TRYPANOSOMES

Pages 101–103

On page 278 of Stuart Gilbert's translation of Nobel Prize winner Albert Camus' novel *The Plague* (New York: Alfred A. Knopf, 1948), Camus expresses beautifully how those who deal with animal or plant protection like to feel about themselves as they "strive their utmost to be healers"—why in each of the campaigns men outdid themselves to combat the fly and trypanosomes.

Pages 103–107

The campaign to break man-fly contact by moving people away from fly haunts is based on material from Robert Koch and Winston Churchill, both cited in Chapter II, and from others but particularly Sir Hesketh Bell. The passage below reveals the relative importance Sir Hesketh gave to home leave and to Theodore Roosevelt, who during Bell's administration was big game hunting in East Africa. Sir Hesketh's attitude typified that of many extremely conscientious colonial officers who suffered sickness and inconvenience in the course of their tours of duty. Come presidents hunting trophies or flies bearing sleeping sickness, home leave was home leave and it had to be respected. On pages 203–204 of *Glimpses of a Governor's Life* (London: Sampson Low, Marston, 1946), Sir Hesketh wrote:

"18*th March* [1908].

"President Roosevelt, with his son Kermit and a party, are now in East Africa shooting. They are coming on here shortly but, as I am going Home, I fear I will not be here to greet them.

"I received yesterday a very interesting letter from the great man. He must have typed it himself, and it is evident that he is a beginner at the machine. The screed is full of amusing mistakes and erasures and almost devoid of punctuation. In one part of it he says: 'I would like to get a good big elephant and a white rhino if possible. Where is the chief missionary center?' I am going to tell him that he ought to get a good tusker in Buddu and a white rhino near Wadelai, but that there is a 'close season,' all the year round, for missionaries."

Pages 163 and 164 of this work provided the material quoted in the text about his meeting in London with Sir Patrick Manson and others; page 167, his description of Churchill's arrival in Uganda.

The absorptive capacity of Churchill's mind as he described his first impressions of Uganda and the grasp he had of strategy even as he directed attention toward what to do about a lowly fly are clearly evident in *My African Journey* (New York and London: Hodder and Stoughton, 1908). His statement about the "fine-spun net being woven remorselessly" around the tsetse fly is found on page 102 of that work; other quotations are from page v of the Preface and from pages 86, 90, and 94 of the text.

Pages 107–124

Príncipe Island intrigued me for several reasons. Despite the lack of general historical information about Príncipe, it would make a marvelous subject for study in its own right as an isolated geographical reception center for a variety of peoples—how they adjusted to each other and related to their parent stock in their original homelands. Moreover, for a woman in the early nineteenth century to have owned virtually a whole island in tropical waters for reasons poorly understood is exciting in itself and arouses one's curiosity. Finally, Príncipe offered a classical, thoroughly documented case for the eradication strategy as applied to tsetse and trypanosomes; the surrounding sea was a geographical barrier, that made it nearly impossible to reintroduce the vector and its disease as eradication measures were in progress.

For historical background on Portugal and her African colonies, I relied mostly on R. J. Hammond's *Portugal and Africa, 1815–1910* (Stanford: Stanford University Press, 1966), and James Duffy's *Portugal in Africa* (Baltimore: Penguin, 1963). The nineteenth-century descriptions of Príncipe come from Volume II of William Allen and T. R. H. Thomson's two-volume *A Narrative of the Expedition Sent by Her Majesty's Government to the River Niger in 1841* (London: Richard Bentley, 1848) and from Thomas J. Hutchinson's *Narrative of the Niger, Tshadda, and Binuë Exploration* . . . (London, 1855; reprinted London: Frank Cass, 1966). The quotation about St. Antonio is from page 189 of the latter work, those describing West Bay, Príncipe, and Madame Ferreira from pages 34 to 36 of the former. The 1841 expedition suffered high mortality, largely because orders to use quinine were not always followed; the 1854–1855 expedition made medical history because under official orders quinine was used as a prophylactic and there was no mortality at all—which convinced Europeans that they could, after all, live in Africa.

While the 1911–1914 tsetse campaign was still on, Bernardo Francisco Bruto da Costa wrote *Sleeping Sickness in the Island of Principe*, translated by J. A. Wyllie (London: Baillière, Tindall and Cox for the Centro Colonial, Lisbon, 1913). The description of Príncipe as "a colossal bouquet of greenery" comes from page 55 of B. F. Bruto da Costa *et al.*, *Sleeping Sickness: A Record of Four Years' War against It in Principe, Portuguese West Africa*, translated by J. A. Wyllie (London: Baillière, Tindall and Cox for the Centro Colonial, Lisbon, 1916). Bruto da Costa also discussed the campaigns in his autobiography, *Vinte e Três Anos ao Serviço do País no Combate às Doenças—África* (Lisbon: Depositária Livraria Portugalia, 1939). Volume I of H. Harold Scott's *A History of Tropical Medicine* (London: Edward Arnold, 1939) likewise contains an extensive discussion of the Príncipe campaigns.

A. G. Gardiner in his *Life of George Cadbury* (London and New York: Cassell, 1923) described the boycott against cacao from

Príncipe Island; some question exists as to the actual efficacy of the boycott, however.

The report of the first Portuguese commission, in French, provides a convenient summary of observations of sleeping sickness in Portugal's West African territories and elsewhere. It is Annibal Bettencourt *et al.*, *La Maladie du sommeil: Rapport présenté au Ministère de la Marine et des Colonies* . . . (Lisbon: Imprimerie de Libanio da Silva, 1903).

The report of the death of Mariana Manoel from sleeping sickness in 1859 is from page 125 and several short quotations about the reappearance of tsetse on Príncipe Island in the 1950's are from pages 131 to 133 of João Fraga de Azevedo *et al.*, *O Reaparecimento da* Glossina palpalis palpalis *na Ilha do Príncipe* (*The Reappearance of* Glossina palpalis palpalis *in Principe Island*) (Lisbon: Junta de Investigações do Ultramar, 1961; Estudos, Ensaios e Documentos No. 89) in Portuguese and English, which is the principal work on the episode.

References to Harris and Morris traps and their uses will be found in the notes to a subsequent section of this chapter.

Pages 124–134

Virginia Thompson and Richard Adloff are the authors of two comprehensive works, both published by the Stanford University Press: *French West Africa* (Stanford, 1958) and *The Emerging States of French Equatorial Africa* (Stanford, 1960). André Gide, in his famous *Travels in the Congo* (*Voyage au Congo* and *Le Retour du Tchad*, Paris: Gallimard, 1927 and 1928) translated Dorothy Bussy (Berkeley and Los Angeles, University of California Press, 1957), graphically describes the ravages of sleeping sickness in French Africa during the 1920's.

I have depended mostly on Albert Schweitzer's own writings to describe his work, and I have quoted directly from his books: *On the Edge of the Primeval Forest and More from the Primeval Forest* (New York: Macmillan, 1948), and *Out of My Life and Thought: An Autobiography*, translated by C. T. Campion (New York: Henry Holt, 1949). Page 4 of the latter book is the source of the quotation concerning his fascination in mastering subjects in which he lacked talent; page 114 of the statement regarding his offer to the Paris Missionary Society. N'Tsama's comment that the doctor was his father is found on page 204 of *On the Edge of the Primeval Forest.* From page 233 of *Out of My Life and Thought* comes Schweitzer's statement that he rejoices over "new remedies" for sleeping sickness; from page 156, his account of how the phrase "Reverence for Life" flashed into his mind; and from page 261, his report that "the Government has taken over the fight against sleeping sickness." The obituary in the September 6, 1965, *New York Times* has also been useful.

M. Marcel Bebey-Eyidi's *La Vie et l'oeuvre médico-sociale en Afrique intertropicale française d'Eugène Jamot (1879–1937)* (Roanne: Imp. Sully, 1950; Faculté de Médecine de Paris: Thèse pour le Doctorat en Médecine, 1950, No. 360), an excellent biography, is probably more laudatory than it need be of Jamot and his work, but it is a crucial reference. Besides this thesis, a useful obituary of Jamot appeared in *Bulletin de la Société de Pathologie Exotique* 30 (5): 337–340, 1937, and a memorial article by H. de Marqueissac in *Biologie Médicale,* 44 (1): 1–4, January, 1955. E. Roubaud's "Les précurseurs dans la lutte contre la maladie du sommeil en Afrique Noire française (1908–1930)," *Presse Médicale,* 63 (75): 1547–1548, November 12, 1955, is important for its treatment of workers who preceded Jamot as well as for Jamot himself. In "La maladie du sommeil il y a 30 ans," *Presse Médicale,* 63 (45): 947–948, June 18, 1955, Henri Galiard said, "La carrière africaine de Jamot est un poème épique."

In English there is a translation from French of an essay by A. J. Lotte entitled "Eugene Jamot's contribution to the success of mobile teams" (Geneva: World Health Organization, 1955; WHO/VDT/146). Lotte is also the author of "The prophylaxis of sleeping sickness in aquatic regions" published in International Scientific Committee for Trypanosomiasis Research, *Fifth Meeting, Pretoria, 1954* (Leopoldville: Permanent Inter-African Bureau for Tsetse and Trypanosomiasis, 1954; B.P.I.T.T. Publication No. 206, English texts), pp. 29–35. The paper preceding this in the same

274 BIBLIOGRAPHICAL ESSAY AND NOTES

publication is also of interest: A. Masseguin and J. Taillefer-Grimaldi, "Statistical review of trypanosomiasis in French West Africa from 1932 to 1954," *ibid.*, 1–25. K. R. S. Morris, the author of a number of articles on the epidemiology of sleeping sickness, has discussed the area in question and the influence of Jamot and his work in "Focal nature of an epidemic disease," *Nature* 193 (4820): 1022–1024, March 17, 1962; "The movement of sleeping sickness across central Africa," *Journal of Tropical Medicine and Hygiene* 66 (3): 59–76, March 1963; and "New frontiers to health in Africa," *Science* 132 (3428): 652–658, September 9, 1960.

Finally, mention should be made of some of Eugene Jamot's own papers: "Essai de prophylaxie médicale de la maladie du sommeil dans l'Oubangui-Chari," *Bulletin de la Société de Pathologie Exotique* 13: 343–375, 1920; "État sanitaire et dépopulation au Congo," *ibid.*, 127–138, 1920; and "La maladie du sommeil au Cameroun," *Bulletin de la Société de Pathologie Exotique* 18: 762–769, 1925; and Letonturier, de Marqueissac, and Jamot, "Essai du tryparsamide dans la trypanosomiase humaine à virus gambiense," *Bulletin de la Société de Pathologie Exotique* 17: 692–703, 1924.

The quotation characterizing Schweitzer as a man of action comes from John Gunther's *Inside Africa* (New York: Harper, 1955), page 724, and the one ascribing a philosophical nature to Jamot is from the Bebey-Eyidi thesis (1950), page 23.

Pages 134–156

Three successive generations of the Swynnerton family have served Britain with distinction abroad. The Reverend Charles Swynnerton collected and edited a volume on Indian folklore, *Romantic Tales from the Panjâb, with Illustrations by Native Hands* (Westminster: Archibald Constable, 1903). Charles F. M. Swynnerton, the central figure of this section, became well known as a naturalist and entomologist; Roger Swynnerton, living in England today, implemented in Kenya the Swynnerton plan, a system of organized small holdings for African farmers that enjoyed brilliant success.

For my characterization of C. F. M. Swynnerton, I have drawn heavily on personal communications from Professor John F. V. Phillips and on the unpublished memoirs of Major H. C. Stiebel entitled "The Tanganyika I Knew"—the latter with the kind permission of Major Stiebel's son and daughter-in-law—and I have made use of some observations by C. F. M.'s son Roger Swynnerton, Dr. T. A. M. Nash, and Dr. Hugh Bunting. For information by Swynnerton on his early studies of the fly see "An examination of the tsetse problem in North Mossurise, Portuguese East Africa," *Bulletin of Entomological Research* 11 (4): 315–385, March 1921; "An experiment in control of tsetse-flies at Shinyanga, Tanganyika Territory," *Bulletin of Entomological Research* 15 (4): 313–337, April 1925; and "How forestry may assist towards the control of the tsetse flies," in R. S. Troup, *Colonial Forest Administration* (London: Oxford University Press, 1940), pp. 439–442. Those interested in Swynnerton's writings on birds and butterflies will be able to find some titles in the biography of him published in *Who Was Who, 1929–1940*, pp. 1318–1319.

For detailed information on the species *Glossina swynnertoni,* three articles may be of interest: E. E. Austen, "A new East African tsetse-fly (Genus *Glossina,* Wied.), which apparently disseminates sleeping sickness," *Bulletin of Entomological Research* 13 (3): 311–315, January 1923; J. P. Glasgow and E. Bursell, "Seasonal variations in the fat content and size of *Glossina swynnertoni* Austen," *Bulletin of Entomological Research* 51 (4): 705–713, January 1961; and J. P. Glasgow and J. R. Welch, "Long-term fluctuations in numbers of the tsetse fly *Glossina swynnertoni* Austen," *Bulletin of Entomological Research* 53 (1): 129–137, April 1962.

Two of C. F. M. Swynnerton's other writings on tsetse are basic, notably "The entomological aspects of an outbreak of sleeping sickness near Mwanza, Tanganyika Territory," *Bulletin of Entomological Research* 13 (3): 317–370, January 1923, and his book entitled *The Tsetse Flies of East Africa* (London: Royal Entomological Society, 1936; *Transactions of the Royal Entomological Society of London,* Vol. 84), which is an indispensable source.

J. P. Glasgow's "Shinyanga: A review of the work of the tsetse research laboratory," *East African Agricultural and Forestry Journal* 26 (1): 22–34, July 1960, contributes to the understanding of the Shinyanga experiments. Swynnerton's words about the cleansing effect of frequent burns have been quoted from page 32 of this article.

For discussions of sleeping sickness itself, various publications are important. They include P. A. Buxton's official survey of *Trypanosomiasis in Eastern Africa, 1947* (London: HMSO for the Colonial Office, 1948); F. I. C. Apted's "Sleeping sickness in Tanganyika, past, present, and future," *Transactions of the Royal Society of Tropical Medicine and Hygiene* 56 (1): 15–29, January 1962; William H. Dye, "The relative importance of man and beast in human trypanosomiasis," *Transactions of the Royal Society of Tropical Medicine and Hygiene* 21 (3): 187–198, November 1927; and two articles by George Maclean: "The relationship between economic development and Rhodesian sleeping sickness in Tanganyika Territory," *Annals of Tropical Medicine and Parasitology* 23 (1): 37–46, April 26, 1929, and "Sleeping sickness measures in Tanganyika Territory," *Kenya and East African Medical Journal* 7 (5): 120–126, August 1930. H. Fairbairn's article, "The agricultural problems posed by sleeping sickness settlements," *East African Agricultural Journal* 9: 17–22, July 1943, will give the reader a vivid picture of the delicate balance between the population of a disease-bearing vector and that of human beings necessary to engender an epidemic and to keep it going. Human beings either too sparsely or too thickly concentrated can impede the progress of an epidemic. Therein lies a powerful control measure often ignored.

Of interest in relation to Swynnerton's general ecological approach is P. E. Glover's "The importance of ecological studies in the control of tsetse flies," *Bulletin of the World Health Organization* 37: 581–614, 1967.

For the earlier game destruction work at Shinyanga, see H. Harrison's "The Shinyanga game experiment: A few of the early observations," *Journal of Animal Ecology* 5: 271–293, 1936.

For the experiments after Swynnerton's death, see W. H. Potts and C. H. N. Jackson, "The Shinyanga game destruction experiment," *Bulletin of Entomological Research* 43 (2): 365–374, July 1952. J. F. V. Phillips set forth, in a personal communication to me, the quoted statements about the need for livestock control and the "stalemate" assessment of the tsetse fly population in Tanganyika territory.

Pages 156–173

T. A. M. Nash's *The Anchau Rural Development and Settlement Scheme* (London: H.M.S.O. for the Colonial Office, 1948) is the basic source for the Anchau scheme; quotes from pages 6 and 14 describe old Anchau and its residents. A prolific writer, Nash authored several other works which I have used: *Tsetse Flies in British West Africa* (London: H.M.S.O. for the Colonial Office, 1948), and two short articles, both in *Bulletin of Entomological Research* 35 (1), April 1944: "The control of sleeping sickness in the raphia pole trade" (page 49), and "A low density of tsetse flies associated with a high incidence of sleeping sickness" (page 51). One of the companion reports to the two by Nash is T. H. Davey, *Trypanosomiasis in British West Africa* (London, H.M.S.O. for the Colonial Office, 1948).

A wealth of historical and ethnographic material is available on both the Hausa and the Fulani; to list it is beyond the scope of this book, but mention must be made of two works of which I made direct use: the interesting personal history of *Baba of Karo: A Woman of the Muslim Hausa*, edited by M. F. Smith (New York: Philosophical Library, 1955) from page 189 of which comes the quote about collecting the spirits to assure the market's success, and Horace Miner's "Culture change under pressure: A Hausa case," *Human Organization* 19 (3): 164–167, Fall 1960.

Cyprian Ekwensi, the Nigerian novelist who wrote *Burning Grass: A Story of the Fulani of Northern Nigeria* (London and Ibadan: Heinemann Educational Books, 1962), put his finger on the basic reason why the Anchau Rural Development Scheme failed over the long term. It was too perfect, too clean, like the town of "New Chanka," which Ekwensi describes on page 57 of his novel. This fictitious city might well have been New Anchau. Whoever the people, I believe it to be biologically unsound that they should stand an environment too antiseptic.

There is a very comprehensive book by P. E. Glover on *The Tsetse Problem in Northern Nigeria* (Nairobi: Patwa News Agency, 1961). Glover has also provided a good general review of research in his previously mentioned article "The importance of ecological studies in the control of tsetse flies," *Bulletin of the World Health Organization* 37: 581–614, 1967.

A. J. Duggan is the author of a most useful and interesting account, "A survey of sleeping sickness in Northern Nigeria from the earliest times to the present day," *Transactions of the Royal Society of Tropical Medicine and Hygiene* 56: 439–486, November 1962. Further background on the development of the Sleeping Sickness Service can be found in a report by Walter B. Johnson entitled *Notes upon a Journey through Certain Belgian, French and British African Dependencies to Observe General Medical Organisation and Methods of Trypanosomiasis Control* (Lagos: Government Printer, 1929), and in a series of articles by H. M. O. Lester: "Sleeping sickness in Northern Nigeria: A review of events leading to the adoption of present methods" and "The progress of sleeping sickness work in Northern Nigeria," *West African Medical Journal,* 6: 50–53, 1933, and 10: 2–10, 1938, respectively, and "The results of sleeping sickness work in Northern Nigeria" and "Further progress in the control of sleeping sickness in Nigeria," *Transactions of the Royal Society of Tropical Medicine and Hygiene* 32 (5): 615–627, February 1939, and 38 (6): 425–444, July 1945, respectively.

Pages 173–176

Four of the books mentioned in notes to earlier chapters contain material on fly boys and fly rounds: P. A. Buxton's *The Natural History of Tsetse Flies*, T. A. M. Nash's *Africa's Bane*, and C. F. M. Swynnerton's *The Tsetse Flies of East Africa* (all cited in full in the notes for the entomology section of the general works) and P. E. Glover's *The Tsetse Problem in Northern Nigeria*, just cited. Two other books also contain important material on fly rounds:

R. C. Muirhead-Thomson, *Ecology of Insect Vector Populations* (London and New York: Academic Press, 1968), and T. R. E. Southwood, *Ecological Methods, with Particular Reference to the Study of Insect Populations* (London: Methuen, 1966). Nash voiced his recollections of Swedi Abdallah to Miss Widenmann in 1967. Important articles dealing with the subject include two by J. P. Glasgow: "Recent fundamental work on tsetse flies," *Annual Review of Entomology* 12: 421–438, 1967, and "The variability of fly-round catches in field studies of *Glossina*," *Bulletin of Entomological Research* 51 (4): 781–787, January 1961; and K. R. S. Morris, "Problems in the assessment of tsetse populations," *ibid.* 52 (2): 239–256, June 1961.

Pages 176–179

The difficulties of sleeping sickness control in the Sudan are chronicled by, among others, E. E. Evans-Pritchard in the anthropological classic *Witchcraft, Oracles and Magic among the Azande* (Oxford: Clarendon Press, 1937). Also on fly and sleeping sickness control in the Sudan are: H. M. O. Leoter, "Certain aspects of trypanosomiasis in some African dependencies," *Transactions of the Royal Society of Tropical Medicine and Hygiene* 33 (1): 11–36, June 1939; A. R. Hunt and J. F. E. Bloss, "Tsetse fly control and sleeping sickness in the Sudan," *ibid.* 39 (1): 43–58, September 1945; and two articles by Bloss alone: "The history of sleeping sickness in the Sudan," *Proceedings of the Royal Society of Medicine* 53 (6): 421–426, June 1960, and "The tsetse fly in the Sudan," *Sudan Notes and Records* 26: 139–156, 1945. E. Aneurin Lewis has described "Tsetse flies carried by railway trains in Kenya colony," *Bulletin of Entomological Research* 40 (4): 511–531, February 1950.

Pages 179–186

The whole concept of fly trapping is based on a knowledge of what attracts flies and what repels them—especially through their senses of sight and smell. On the use of traps, P. A. Buxton's *The Natural History of Tsetse Flies* (1955) has an extensive treatment.

For Harris traps, see especially two articles by R. H. T. P. Harris, "Some facts and figures regarding the attempted control of *Glossina pallidipes* in Zululand," *South African Journal of Science* 29: 495–507, October 1932; and "The control and possible extermination of the tsetse by trapping," in *Acta Conventus Tertii de Tropicis atque Malariae Morbis* (Amsterdam: Societas Neerlandica Medicinae Tropicae, 1938), I: 663–677. The quotations about the "ten skilled native shots" and the game destroyed being "in the category of vermin" are from page 496 of the first Harris article.

Swynnerton describes many bizarre types of traps in his treatise *The Tsetse Flies of East Africa* (1936). K. R. S. Morris and M. G. Morris go into great detail about their traps in "The use of traps against tsetse in West Africa," *Bulletin of Entomological Research* 39 (4): 491–528, March 1949. This man and wife team could quite as easily and at least as accurately have entitled their article "What people will not do to try to fool a fly." K. R. S. Morris wrote about "Trapping as a means of studying the game tsetse, *Glossina pallidipes* Aust." in the *Bulletin of Entomological Research* 51 (3): 533–556, November 1960. Reference should also be made to a multipart article by I. M. Smith and B. D. Rennison entitled "Studies of the sampling of *Glossina pallidipes* Aust.," which appeared in the *Bulletin of Entomological Research* 52 (1 and 3): 165–189 and 601–619, April and October 1961, especially part four of the article, entitled "Some aspects of the use of Morris traps," pp. 609–619. C. B. Symes's article "Outline of work on *G. palpalis* in Kenya," *East African Medical Journal* 12 (9): 263–281, December 1935, discusses experiments with block trapping, in which scents were used as attractants.

Pages 186–190

For the poison-bait cattle experiments see G. F. Burnett, "The effect of poison bait cattle on populations of *Glossina morsitans* Westw. and *G. swynnertoni* Aust.," *Bulletin of Entomological Research* 45 (3): 411–421, September 1954, and E. F. Whiteside, "An experiment in control of tsetse with DDT-treated oxen," *ibid*. 40 (1): 123–134, May 1949.

The Kibori River spraying program has been described by A. R. Mahood in "The control of *Glossina palpalis* (R.-D.) in the Guinea savannah zone of Northern Nigeria," in International Scientific Committee for Trypanosomiasis Research, *Ninth Meeting, Conakry, 1962* (London, 1963; CCTA, Publication No. 88), pp. 171–179.

Pages 190–197

The Ankole program is discussed in W. R. Wooff's "The eradication of *Glossina morsitans morsitans* Westw. in Ankole, Western Uganda, by dieldrin application," in International Scientific Committee for Trypanosomiasis Research, *Tenth Meeting, Kampala, 1964* ([London], 1965; CCTA, Publication No. 97), pp. 157–166. Dr. Wooff has also discussed his work in personal communications to me.

R. du Toit describes the aerial spraying campaign in Zululand in "Trypanosomiasis in Zululand and the control of tsetse flies by chemical means," *Onderstepoort Journal of Veterinary Research* 26 (3): 317–387, June 1954. An unsigned article entitled "D.D.T. and the aeroplane in the control of the tsetse fly and trypanosomiasis in South Africa," *Nature* 160 (4067): 485–486, October 11, 1947, also deals with this campaign. The East African experiments are documented in a multipart series "Aircraft Applications of Insecticides in East Africa" by various authors from the Colonial Insecticide Research Unit, Arusha, Tanganyika, K. S. Hocking being the senior author of most of the articles, in the *Bulletin of Entomological Research* for 1953 and 1954, Volumes 44 and 45.

Carroll M. Williams' "Third-generation pesticides," *Scientific American* 217 (1): 13–17, July 1967, provides a convenient summary of juvenile hormone and "paper factor." One might also refer to Lawrence Lessing's "A molecular bomb for the war against insects," *Fortune* 78 (1): 86–89, 116, 118, 121, July 1968, E. F. Knipling's "Sterile technique—Principles involved, current application, limitations, and future application," in *Genetics of Insect Vectors of Disease*, edited for the World Health Organization by J. W. Wright and R. Pal (Amsterdam, London, and New York: Elsevier,

1967), pp. 587–616; and David A. Dame, Godfrey J. W. Dean, and John Ford, "Investigations of the sterile male technique with *Glossina moritans,*" in International Scientific Committee for Trypanosomiasis Research, *Tenth Meeting, Kampala, 1964* ([London], 1965; CCTA, Publication No. 97), pp. 93–96.

An article by Dame and Claude H. Schmidt, "The sterile-male technique against tsetse flies, *Glossina* spp.," *Bulletin of the Entomological Society of America* 16 (1): 24–30, March 1970, may well be the standard reference on the subject for some time to come.

Pages 197–206

The lines from Act IV, Scene 1, of Shakespeare's *The Tragedy of Macbeth,* quoted from pages 63 and 64 of the Yale Shakespeare revised edition of this work edited by Eugene M. Waith (New Haven: Yale University Press, 1954; London: Geoffrey Cumberlege, Oxford University Press, 1954), portray a trial and error technique also characteristic of even so exact a science as we think modern chemistry to be when applied to the delicate matter of searching for drugs to combat trypanosomes in the bloodstream. The Livingstones' description of their encounter with the Batoka chief's son, which is found on page 233 of *Narrative of an Expedition to the Zambesi . . .* (London: John Murray, 1865), constitutes another example; and the sequence from "B.C." which appeared in the *New York Herald Tribune* (Paris edition) for February 6–7, 1965, and which is reproduced here by kind permission of John Hart and Field Enterprises, Inc., is the third allusion to the role of chance or luck in research.

In the text I have not dwelt on dietary abnormalities that may accompany sleeping sickness although evidence seems to suggest that geophagy (eating of earth) and craving for meat occur with the disease. David Livingstone's encounters with geophagy are described in Michael Gelfand's *Livingstone the Doctor* (Oxford: Basil Blackwell, 1957). Geophagy in cattle and its connection with trypanosomiasis are discussed by P. E. Glover in *The Tsetse Problem in Northern Nigeria* (1961), and the craving of sleeping sickness patients for meat, in part 1 of J. N. P. Davies's "The cause of sleeping sickness?," *East African Medical Journal* 39 (3): 81–99, March 1962.

The fascinating story of quinine in the prevention and cure of malaria has been told many times. An interesting account of the acceptance of the drug may be found in Philip Curtin's *The Image of Africa* (Madison: University of Wisconsin Press, 1964). Paul F. Russell brings the story to mid-twentieth century in *Man's Mastery of Malaria* (London and New York: Oxford University Press, 1955).

The "Paul Ehrlich Centennial," *Annals of the New York Academy of Sciences* 59 (2): 141–276, September 23, 1954, furnishes extensive material about Paul Ehrlich and his role in the development of chemotherapy, especially in contributions by C. H. Browning and Hugo Bauer. Browning is also the author of another useful two-part article: "Emil Behring and Paul Ehrlich: Their contributions to science," *Nature* 175 (4457): 570–575, April 2, 1955, and 175 (4458): 616–619, April 9, 1955.

H. Wolferstan Thomas and Anton Breinl discussed their investigations in *Report on Trypanosomes, Trypanosomiasis, and Sleeping Sickness* . . . (London: Williams and Norgate for the University Press of Liverpool, 1905; Liverpool School of Tropical Medicine, Memoir XVI).

What I have said about tryparsamide is based chiefly on George W. Corner, *A History of the Rockefeller Institute, 1901–1953* (New York: Rockefeller Institute Press, 1964), and Louise Pearce, "Tryparsamide treatment of African sleeping sickness," *Science* 61 (1569): 90–92, January 23, 1925. Pearce's article refers to field work by the French as well as to her own investigations.

Ernst A. H. Friedheim's "Some approaches to the development of chemotherapeutic compounds," *Annals of Tropical Medicine and Parasitology* 53 (1): 1–9, April 1959, is particularly readable, and I have made extensive use of it. Other especially useful works are James Williamson's "Chemotherapy and chemoprophylaxis of African trypanosomiasis," *Experimental Parasitology* 12 (4): 274–322, August 1962, and 12 (5): 323–367, October 1962, and

James Grier's *A History of Pharmacy* (London: Pharmaceutical Press, 1937).

The article by Friedheim referred to above provides a good summary of the studies he conducted with the melarsens but was published before the development of Mel W. One article on that substance is H. J. C. Watson, "Final report on a field trial of Mel. W. in the treatment of Gambian sleeping sickness," in International Scientific Committee for Trypanosomiasis Research, *Tenth Meeting, Kampala, 1964* ([London], 1965; CCTA, Publication No. 97), pp. 193–195. Friedheim has reported on another substance in "Mel D: A possible alternative to Mel W," *Transactions of the Royal Society of Tropical Medicine and Hygiene* 64 (1): 163–164, 1970.

R. E. Duxbury and E. H. Sadun working at Walter Reed Army Institute of Research, Washington, D.C., have reported on "Resistance produced in mice and rats by inoculation with irradiated *Trypanosoma rhodesiense*," *Journal of Parasitology* 55 (4): 859–865, August 1969.

On immunology, one must refer to A. R. Gray, widely recognized as an authority in this field, "The epidemiological significance of some recent findings from research on antigenic variation in trypanosomes," *Bulletin of the World Health Organization* 41 (6): 805–813, 1969. One might also wish to consult P. G. Cunnington's "Immunization of rats with a series of consecutive relapse variants of *Trypanosoma brucei*," *Transactions of the Royal Society of Tropical Medicine and Hygiene* 64 (1): 169, 1970; W. H. R. Lumsden's "The estimation of the concentration of the IgM class of immunoglobulins in the serum as an aid to the diagnosis of trypanosomiasis in man," in International Scientific Committee for Trypanosomiasis Research, *Tenth Meeting, Kampala 1964* ([London], 1965; CCTA, Publication No. 97), pp. 203–204, and a number of articles by M. P. Cunningham.

CHAPTER IV—"YOU TELL ME TO SIT QUIET"

Pages 207–210

I chose the title and excerpts from Archibald Campbell Jordan's poem "You tell me to sit quiet," published in *Poems from Black*

Africa, edited by Langston Hughes (Bloomington: Indiana University Press, 1963), pp. 111–113, to express the current of my thought in this chapter on man's relationship to the fly today because his poem strikes at three of the most important forces shaping Africa—educating the masses, forming leadership, and building nations. One can speculate that lifting the curse that tsetse flies and their trypanosomes imposed on Africa made these objectives attainable. The excerpts are used with the permission of the publisher.

The reader will recognize two additional themes in this chapter —first, the suspicion with which the man of action usually views the ivy-towered research worker and vice versa; second, the tremendous shake-up in programs and institutions devoted to scientific endeavor which political and economic changes on the continent of Africa have wrought. Nation-building especially during the decade of the sixties forced a real test of the sort of research African people are prepared to support.

One of the grand old men of action in tsetse and trypanosome control operations of French-speaking Africa, P. Richet, articulated "to prevent men dying" as the most important aim of their efforts in *Control and Surveillance Techniques in Human Trypanosomiasis* (Geneva: WHO Expert Committee on Trypanosomiasis, 1962; WHO/Tryp/34), p. 2. Ernst A. H. Friedheim, who developed Mel W and Mel B for sleeping sickness treatment, knew Richet quite well. In conversation with me he attributed to Richet a single-handed success in carrying the French program for sleeping sickness control from a cohesive one in colonial days through a shattered program when independence came to a cohesive one again in recent years by virtue of his personality and his ability diplomatically to get people to work together. He also remembered Richet, a general with all possible stars, out hunting in an open-necked shirt and baggy pants, or garbed in "bikini"-type shorts and sneakers.

Virginia Thompson and Richard Adloff in *The Emerging States of French Equatorial Africa* (Stanford: Stanford University Press, 1960), page 331, refer to the early explorers of French Equatorial Africa, notably Noël Ballay and Emile Gentil and the latter's gift for an institute in Brazzaville, but for additional information about these men one must consult *Le Grand Larousse encyclopédique*

(1962) and *Larousse du XXe siècle* (1958). The *Encyclopaedia Britannica*, 11th ed. (1911), 11: 101, gives further information about Ballay and Gentil in an historical account of the French Congo.

Pages 210–216

H. Harold Scott in Volume I of *A History of Tropical Medicine* (1939) has given a panoramic account of the many commissions that European governments and schools of tropical medicine organized to investigate the sleeping sickness problem. R. L. Sheppard, who joined the Sleeping Sickness Bureau in 1910, described its founding and early history in "Tropical Diseases Bulletin, Volume Fifty," *Tropical Diseases Bulletin* 50 (1): 1–2, January 1953.

To appreciate the extent to which flies and trypanosomes aroused concern and stimulated research on a truly international scale one must read, in addition to perusing Scott's historical accounts in *A History of Tropical Medicine* (1939), the publications of the Health Organisation of the League of Nations. Their publications most useful in this regard include those of the Expert Committee of the League of Nations Health Committee: Andrew Balfour *et al.*, *Interim Report on Tuberculosis and Sleeping-Sickness in Equatorial Africa* ([Geneva], 1923; C.8.M.6. 1924. III) and A. Balfour *et al.*, *Further Report on Tuberculosis and Sleeping-Sickness in Equatorial Africa* (Geneva, 1925; C.H. 281) and *Final Report of the League of Nations International Commission on Human Trypanosomiasis* (Geneva, 1928; C.H. 629). These three voluminous papers constituted the last word in research, particularly on the trypanosomes, through the 1920's. A subsequent *Report of the Second International Conference on Sleeping-Sickness Held in Paris November 5th to 7th, 1928* (Geneva: League of Nations, 1928; C.H. 743) gives important information on sleeping sickness in the Sudan; it also presents material from Togoland, Cameroon, Morocco, Spanish Guinea, and Fernando Po in addition to recommendations regarding the manner in which the Health Organisation of the League of Nations might assist in coordinating investigations on sleeping sickness.

Edgar B. Worthington's text on *Science in the Development of Africa* published in London by the Commission for Technical Cooperation in Africa South of the Sahara and the Scientific Council for Africa South of the Sahara in 1958 is a good source of information about these organizations known as CCTA/CSA. In this text he also describes the organization of the Bureau Permanent Interafricain pour la Tsé-Tsé et la Trypanosomiase (BPITT) and the development simultaneously of the International Scientific Committee, later Council, for Trypanosomiasis Research (ISCTR). Subsequent to Worthington's book, reports from the biennial meetings of CSA and of ISCTR offer information on the growth and development of these organizations and on BPITT. Scientific Council for Africa, *Fourteenth Meeting of the Scientific Council, Lagos, 1964* (London, 1964; CCTA Publication No. 92), and International Scientific Committee for Trypanosomiasis Research, *Tenth Meeting, Kampala, 1964* ([London], 1965; CCTA, Publication No. 97), carry articles explaining BPITT's demise, CCTA's becoming an organ of the Organisation of African Unity (OAU), and the continuing role ISCTR would play as an independent organization. The thirteenth meeting of ISCTR was held in Lagos, Nigeria, in 1971.

Dr. Lucien Raynaud's philosophy can be found in the League of Nations Health Committee *Minutes, 8th Session* (Geneva, 1926; C.610.M.238. 1926), pp. 72–76, in C.H. 510 (1), his "Report on the practicability and desirability of establishing a centre of epidemiological information for the African continent, with provisional headquarters at Algiers."

"Research on tsetse fly and disease," *Nature* 154 (3914): 573, November 4, 1944, tells of the organization of the Tsetse Fly and Trypanosomiasis Committee formed to advise the Colonial Office of Great Britain; it set the stage for building "splendid institutes" for research on these problems in Africa, which to some extent provided homes in Africa for the teams of researchers from the metropolitan countries. T. M. Leach's *Annual Report: 1966* of the Nigerian Institute for Trypanosomiasis Research, formerly the West African Institute for Trypanosomiasis Research, has an historical note that covers the founding and growth of that institute. The creation of its companion institute, the East African Trypanosomiasis Research Organization, is well described by M. A. Soltys in "Golden jubilee of the discovery of sleeping sickness in East Africa," *East African Medical Journal* 30 (9): 389–392, September 1953.

Pages 216–225

In *An African Survey, Revised 1956* (London and New York: Oxford University Press, 1957) on pages 251–254 introducing the section on "The Rising Spirit of Africanism," Lord Hailey gives a concise appraisal of the underlying factors that led the present nations of Africa to achieve independence in rapid succession after World War II and, if one extrapolates, the basis for the crumbling research empire as it relates to the tsetse fly and to trypanosomiasis.

Miss Elizabeth A. Widenmann, who has served as my research assistant throughout the process of writing this book, interviewed T. A. M. Nash in his laboratories at Bristol. I have relied heavily on the copious notes that she took during the day that she spent with him. W. H. R. Lumsden has contributed to an understanding of the problems inherent in conducting research and building research institutions in Africa through his article "Changing patterns of trypanosomiasis research in East Africa," *Transactions of the Royal Society of Tropical Medicine and Hygiene* 58 (2): 97–135, March 1964.

Thomas R. Odhiambo, Director for Scientific Affairs of the International Centre of Insect Physiology and Ecology, warns of certain difficulties African people face in accepting science as being essential for development in his article "East Africa: Science for Development," *Science* 158 (3803): 876–881, November 17, 1967. In line with a major theme of this chapter, he emphasizes the need not simply for Africans to accept technology but also to establish basic scientific research to undergird technology.

Pages 225–238

Joy Adamson makes frequent allusions to the fly, tsetse, in her lion books: *Born Free* (New York: Pantheon Books, 1960), *Living*

Free (New York: Harcourt, Brace and World, 1961), and *Forever Free* (New York: Harcourt, Brace and World, 1963).

Evidence of the impact the fly and sleeping sickness may have had on music, drama, dance, and other social and cultural activities seems singularly wanting in the past literature of Africa. However, in a personal communication to me on December 11, 1971, Dr. Evans D. Offori gave both the Ewe and the English words of two proverbs we had discussed earlier and interpreted them for me. The one about blood in the head of tsetse, I have used in the text. About the other *"Adzoe dze xa nu menyafona o"* (It is difficult to kill a tsetse fly when it is resting on a broom), Dr. Offori explained that the traditional way to kill a tsetse fly is to swat it with a broom, but if it were already on the broom obviously this would be difficult to do without its flying away. He explained further: "Suppose you were a police officer in New York City checking on parking violation; suddenly you find your own car conspicuously parked in a 'no parking' zone say by your wife. Do you give a ticket or let it go? However you look at it, the decision is a difficult one to take." An amulet used against sleeping sickness forms part of the collection of such artifacts in the Wellcome Museum in London and constitutes another bit of evidence of people's awareness of the disease, at least, from early times.

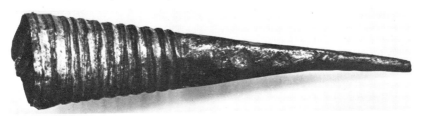

Amulet to ward off sleeping sickness. Shown two-thirds actual size. (Photograph from the Wellcome Historical Museum and Library.)

In modern times and on a somewhat superficial plane tsetse's name has spread far and wide: it enters into international parlance. The bartender in a television show pretended that he had a jacket made of tsetse flies not long ago. A choir director of a college conservatory of music used tsetse as a test combination of syllables to get his trainees to enunciate properly. Ogden Nash has quipped about tsetse in his verse. We have already seen that John Hart has used tsetse as an ingredient for suicide soup in one of his "B.C." cartoons.

Both tsetse and trypanosomes have graced elegant Christmas cards issued by the trypanosomiasis research institute in Nigeria; the nicest one showed the institute's seal in red encircling an engraved trypanosome in gold.

American author Samuel Clemens, French novelist Albert Camus, and African poet Archibald Campbell Jordan, each in his own way called attention to the marvelous comeback quality any species—whether fly, bacterium, or human being—possesses under pressure to survive, as the quotations at the beginnings of Chapter I and Chapter III and the title of Chapter IV imply. Harold Oldroyd, entomologist, who knew Major Austen and other early tsetse fly researchers, articulates this universal quality of a species in describing tsetse as a relic from the past fighting back in his fascinating text *The Natural History of Flies* (New York: W. W. Norton, 1965), p. 280, which I think any layman will enjoy reading. The description of the recrudescence of sleeping sickness around the shores of Lake Victoria is drawn largely from G. R. Barnley, "Resettlement in the South Busoga sleeping sickness area," *East African Medical Journal* 45 (5): 263–265, May 1968.

Other interesting and relatively recent articles which might be noted here include D. M. Blair, E. Burnett Smith, and Michael Gelfand, "Human trypanosomiasis in Rhodesia—New hypothesis suggested for the rarity of human trypanosomiasis," *Central African Journal of Medicine,* supplement to 14 (7), July 1968, 12 pp., and related correspondence, in *ibid.* 14 (9): 208–209, September 1968, and 14 (11): 263–266, November 1968; D. A. T. Baldry, "Variations in the ecology of *Glossina* spp.," *Bulletin of the World Health Organization* 40: 859–869, 1969; and John Ford, "Control of the African trypanosomiases with special reference to land use," *ibid.* 40: 879–892, 1969.

The story about Mr. and Mrs. William T. Davis appeared in the *New York Times,* September 7, 1969. S. K. K. Seah of Queen Mary Veterans Hospital, Montreal, and Sima Gabrielian of Montreal Chinese Hospital gave a clinical description of African trypanosomiasis in the two Canadian volunteers in a note dated July 20, 1972, which was published in *Transactions of the Royal Society of Tropical Medicine and Hygiene* 66 (5): 807, 1972.

The January 1967 issue of the WHO magazine, *World Health,* on page 13 in an item entitled "Sleeping sickness returns" records the figures that support the reference to sleeping sickness reaching rock bottom in 1960 in the Democratic Republic of the Congo (now Zaire) and its subsequent increase. M. P. Hutchinson relates in full the problem of "Human trypanosomiasis in south-west Ethiopia (March 1967–March 1970)," *Ethiopian Medical Journal* 9 (1): 3–69, 1971.

One can cite equally impressive figures of localized outbreaks in other areas of Africa. The World Health Organization issued *Expert Committee on Trypanosomiasis: First Report* (Geneva, 1962; WHO Technical Report Series, No. 247), which summarizes incidence of human and animal trypanosomiasis in many of the tropical countries of Africa as of the late 1950's and early 1960's.

Another important source for statistics especially for 1959 through 1968 is WHO's "Trypanosomiasis in Africa and America," *World Health Statistics Report* 22 (11): 635–703, 1969. Also indispensable for current information are the annual trypanosomiasis roundups published each May in *Tropical Diseases Bulletin* and recent reports of the meetings of the International Scientific Council for Trypanosomiasis Research, now published under the auspices of the Organisation of African Unity.

Finally, I would like to point out that much of the literature on tsetse flies and sleeping sickness cited above is far more interesting than the nature of the titles and the scientific character of the articles would lead one to believe. Every so often, human elements emerge from the description of the research and the reporting of results that lead me to think of an anecdote about education and superstition written by John Scott in the Headline Series of the

Foreign Policy Association booklet, *Africa: World's Last Frontier* (New York, 1959; No. 135), page 7: "We were walking through the market place of the little Senegalese town of M'Bour when I noticed some fingernail-sized pouches tied to the arm of a ten-year-old boy watching us. 'They are *gris-gris,*' said our guide, a government photographer with more university education than I have, 'they protect him from evil.' When I asked whether he believed in *gris-gris,* our guide shrugged. 'As an educated man, I of course cannot believe in these superstitions. On the other hand, as a man of sense, I cannot completely ignore them.' "

In my story about man against tsetse an analogy exists in the personification of tsetse and, on occasion, in imputing purpose to the fly for its actions—thoughts just as antagonistic to science as superstition is to education. Accepting them, however, one strives of course for the highest degree of objective scientific research.

Index

MAN AGAINST TSETSE
STRUGGLE FOR AFRICA

Designed by R. E. Rosenbaum.
Composed by Vail-Ballou Press, Inc., in 10 point linofilm Times Roman, 2 points leaded, with display lines in Helvetica.
Printed offset by Vail-Ballou Press on Warren's Patina II, 60 pound basis.
Bound by Vail-Ballou Press in Columbia book cloth and stamped in All Purpose foil.

Library of Congress Cataloging in Publication Data
(Prepared by the CIP Project for library cataloging purposes only)

McKelvey, John J
    Man against tsetse.

    Bibliography: p.
    1. Trypanosomiasis—Africa.   2. Tsetse flies—Control—Africa.   I. Title.   [DNLM: 1. Trypanosomiasis, African.   2. Tsetse flies.   QX505 M154m 1973]
RC186.T82M3   614.4'322   72-12409
ISBN 0-8014-0768-0